3rd Australian Edition

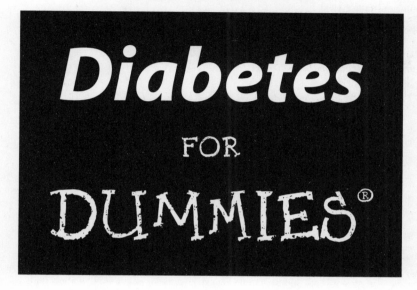

Diabetes FOR DUMMIES®

**Professor Lesley Campbell
and The Diabetes Centre
of St Vincent's Hospital, Sydney
Alan L Rubin, MD**

WILEY

Wiley Publishing Australia Pty Ltd

Diabetes For Dummies®, 3rd Australian edition

Published by
Wiley Publishing Australia Pty Ltd
42 McDougall Street
Milton, Qld 4064
www.dummies.com

Copyright © 2011 Wiley Publishing Australia Pty Ltd

The moral rights of the authors have been asserted.

National Library of Australia
Cataloguing-in-Publication data

Author:	Campbell, Lesley
Title:	Diabetes For Dummies / Lesley Campbell
Edition	3rd Australian edition
ISBN:	978 0 73037 500 5 (pbk.)
Notes:	Includes index
Subjects:	Diabetes — popular works
	Patient education
	Diabetes in children
	Diabetes — Diet therapy
Dewey Number:	994

Cover image: © Ashaki, 2010, Used under license from Shutterstock.com

Typeset by diacriTech, Chennai, India

Printed in China by
Printplus Limited

10 9 8 7 6 5 4 3 2 1

About the Authors

Professor Lesley Campbell, MBBS FRCP (UK) FRACP AM, is the Director of the Diabetes Centre and Services at St Vincent's Hospital, a Professor of Medicine at the University of NSW, a Senior Researcher at the Garvan Institute of Medical Research and a Senior Physician in clinical practice at St Vincent's Hospital. Her research focuses on type 2 diabetes mellitus and obesity. She is specifically interested in the role of central body fat and the genetic factors predisposing to insulin resistance syndrome and type 2 diabetes.

The **Diabetes Centre** at St Vincent's Hospital in Sydney was established in 1982 to promote greater knowledge about diabetes and optimise its management. The centre is a public specialist health service, staffed by a diabetes specialist, a registrar, diabetes educators and dietitian. It also draws on services including private diabetes specialists, general practitioners, podiatrists, ophthalmologists, psychologists and other health professionals. The aim of the Diabetes Centre's multidisciplinary approach is to help people with diabetes to manage their diabetes on a day-to-day basis and to facilitate and co-ordinate the medical, educational and nutritional resources that they need.

Alan L Rubin, MD, is one of America's foremost experts on diabetes. He is a professional member of the American Diabetes Association and the Endocrine Society and has been in private practice specialising in diabetes and thyroid disease for over 25 years.

Authors' Acknowledgements

Acknowledgments from Professor Lesley Campbell

I want to take this opportunity to thank all those who have contributed to this third Australian edition of *Diabetes for Dummies*. My gratitude goes to Melissa Armstrong, who was the main driver in getting this book into production and finally to print. I also want to thank the following people who helped with certain sections of the book: Professor Don Chisholm from the Garvan Institute for Medical Research, Sydney; Dr Jerry Greenfield, Chairman of the Department of Endocrinology at St Vincent's Hospital, Sydney; Dr Paul Lee, Endocrinology Doctoral Candidate from the Garvan Insitute for Medical Research; Jane Ludington, Clinical Pharmacist from St Vincent's Hospital and the University of Sydney; Dr Louise Maple-Brown from the Menzies School of Health Research in Darwin; Dr Gabrielle O'Kane, Microbiologist/Registrar in Diabetes at St Vincent's Hospital; Dr Ann Poynton, Endocrinologist from Prince of Wales Hospital, Sydney; Dr Vanessa Tsang from Royal North Shore Hospital, Sydney; Dr Daniel Chen, Registrar in Endocrinology at St Vincent's Hospital; Dr Kay Wilhelm and Joanna Crawford from the Urban Mental Health Research Institute St Vincent's Hospital; Dr Weng Sam, Visiting Medical Officer, Department of Endocrinology at St Vincent's Hospital; and Karen Jameson, Diabetes Educator at Royal North Shore Hospital in Sydney.

This third edition would not have been possible without the help of the staff at the Diabetes Centre at St Vincent's Hospital in Sydney. I again thank Melissa Armstrong and also Kylie Alexander, Jan Alford, Wendy Bryant, Cathy Carty, Josie Maguire and Penny Morris.

Acknowledgments from Doctor Alan Rubin

I want to thank ophthalmologist Dr John Norris of Pacific Eye Associates in San Francisco for helping me to see the place of the eye physician in diabetes care. I also want to thank podiatrist Dr Mark Pinter for helping me get a leg-up on his specialty. Librarians Mary Ann Zaremska and Nancy Phelps at St Francis Memorial Hospital were tremendously helpful in providing the articles and books upon which the information in the book is based.

My teachers are too numerous to mention, but one group deserves special attention. They are my patients over the last 26 years, the people whose trials and tribulations caused me to seek the knowledge that you will find in this book.

Dedication

We dedicate this book to the people with diabetes whom we have met over the years who have taught us so much and from whom we are still learning — Prof Lesley Campbell and the St Vincent's Hospital Diabetes Team.

This book is dedicated to my wife, Enid, and my children, Renee and Larry. Their patience, enthusiasm, and encouragement helped to make the writing a real pleasure — Alan L Rubin.

Publisher's Acknowledgements

We're proud of this book; please send us your comments through our online registration form located at http://dummies.custhelp.com.

Some of the people who helped bring this book to market include the following:

Acquisitions, Editorial and Media Development

Project Editor: Charlotte Duff

Acquisitions Editor: Rebecca Crisp

Editorial Manager: Hannah Bennett

Production

Graphics: Wiley Art Studio

Cartoons: Glenn Lumsden

Proofreader: Liz Goodman

Indexer: Karen Gillen

The authors and publisher would like to thank the following copyright holders, organisations and individuals for their permission to reproduce copyright material in this book.

- Page 42 and 43: *Diabetes prevalence in Australia*, Australian Institute of Health and Welfare, 2009, p. 23 and p. 25, Diabetes Series Number 14. Reproduced by permission of Australian Institute of Health and Welfare.

Contents at a Glance

Table of Contents

Introduction

You may be thinking there's certainly nothing lucky about being diagnosed with diabetes; after all, it is a disease, isn't it? And you're right, nothing *is* lucky about the diagnosis, but the people who are diagnosed with diabetes early on in the 21st century are the luckiest group in history.

Those of you with diabetes have a decade or more in which to avoid the long-term complications of this disease. In a sense, a diagnosis of diabetes is both good news and bad news. It is bad news because you have a disease you would happily do without. It is good news if you use it to make some changes in your lifestyle that can not only prevent complications but also help you to live a longer and higher quality of life.

As for developing a sense of humour about it, at times you'll feel like doing anything but laughing. But scientific studies are clear about the benefits of a positive attitude. In a very few words: He who laughs, lasts. Another point is that people learn more and retain more when humour is part of the process.

Our goal is not to trivialise human suffering by being comic about it, but to lighten the burden of a chronic disease by showing that it's not all gloom and doom.

About This Book

The book is not meant to be read from cover to cover — although if you know nothing about diabetes, doing so might be a good approach. This book is your source of information on diabetes and the medical research currently under way into new drugs and techniques. So that you may stay abreast of the latest developments in diabetes care, the book also directs you to the best sources of reliable information on any medical advances that may occur after the publication of this edition.

We have tried to provide you with enough information so that you can make informed decisions about how you can care for yourself when you have diabetes, but always remember that you have your GP and members of your diabetes care team to help you through. You are not alone!

Conventions Used in this Book

Diabetes, as you know, is all about sugar. But sugars come in many types. So health professionals avoid using the words *sugar* and *glucose* interchangeably. In this book (unless we slip up), we use the word glucose rather than sugar.

What You Don't Have to Read

Throughout the book, shaded areas, called sidebars, appear. These sidebars contain material that is interesting but not essential. We hereby give you permission to skip them if the material inside them is of no particular interest to you.

Foolish Assumptions

This book assumes that you know nothing about diabetes. You won't suddenly have to face a term that's not explained and that you've never heard of before. For those of you who already know a lot, we provide more in-depth explanations. You can pick and choose how much you want to know about a subject, but the key points are clearly marked.

How This Book Is Organised

This book is divided into seven parts to help you to find out all you can about the topic of diabetes.

Part I: Dealing with the Onset of Diabetes

To slay the dragon, you have to be able to identify it. This part explains the different types of diabetes and how you get them. In this part, you find out how to deal with the emotional and psychological consequences of the diagnosis and what all those big words mean. You also find out how to prevent the complications of diabetes. We also include a chapter on prevention of type 1 and type 2 diabetes to inform you, among other things, about the latest advances in research in this area. We include a chapter on prediabetes, as well, for those who may be diagnosed with the earliest signs of diabetes.

Part II: How Diabetes Affects Your Body

Few diseases affect every part of the body in the way that diabetes does. If you understand diabetes, you will have a fairly good grasp of how other illnesses can change the state of your health.

In this part, you find out what you need to know about both the short- and long-term complications of diabetes. You also find out about some sexual problems related to diabetes and the problems associated with feet for those with diabetes.

Part III: Living with Diabetes: Your Physical Health

In this part, you discover all the tools available to treat diabetes. You find out about the kinds of tests that you should be doing as well as the tests your doctor should be ordering in order to get a clear picture of your diabetes, what to do about it and how to follow treatment.

You also discover the dietary changes that you need to make to help control your blood glucose and how to get the most out of your exercise routine and medications.

Part IV: Living with Diabetes: Your Mental Health

In this part, you read about why looking after your mental health when you have diabetes is just as important as caring for your physical health. This part helps you recognise how you can become your own worst enemy, and provides tips on how to become, and stay, motivated when making lifestyle changes.

This part also helps you understand more about your diabetes care team members and their roles. Finally, you find out about the huge amount of help out there for you and your family. It's yours for the taking, and you should definitely take advantage of it.

Part V: Special Considerations for Living with Diabetes

The way that diabetes develops is different for each age group. In this part, you discover more about those differences and how to manage them. This part also covers the special considerations created by diabetes before, during and after pregnancy, as well as some of the special economic problems that may confront people with diabetes, relating to jobs and insurance.

Lastly, this part covers all the new developments in diagnosing, monitoring and treating diabetes and helps correct a lot of misinformation about diabetes treatment.

Part VI: The Part of Tens

This part presents some key suggestions — the things you most need to know as well as the things you least want to know. You discover the ten commandments of diabetes care and the myths that confuse many people who have diabetes.

This part also provides a comprehensive list of reputable websites where you can find extra help or information about specific areas of diabetes management.

Part VII: Appendixes

This part of the book contains even more information about diabetes. Here, we cover further information on insulin pumps, including tips to help you decide whether this is the right option for you. We also provide practical exercises and further tips to help improve your mental health. And in case you forget what a term means, you can quickly flip to the handy glossary provided here as well.

Icons Used in This Book

The icons tell you what you must know, what you should know and what you might find interesting but can live without.

This icon marks whenever we tell a story about people with diabetes.

Pay attention when you see this icon; it means the information is essential and you need to be aware of it.

This icon points out when you should see your doctor or a member of your diabetes care team (for example, if your blood glucose level is too high or you need a particular test done).

The information provided here is more complex, so you can skip it if you choose.

Listen up. This icon marks important information that can save you time and energy.

When you see this icon, take note. It warns against potential problems (for example, if you don't treat something).

Part I
Dealing with the Onset of Diabetes

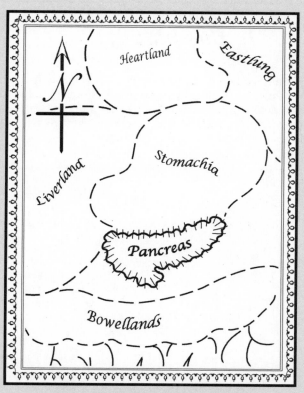

'Pancreas: a small region, often ignored, until it goes on strike.'

In this part . . .

You have been told that you or a loved one has
diabetes. What do you do now? This part helps
you to deal with all the emotions that inevitably arise —
from wondering whether the diagnosis is correct
to investigating the causes of diabetes.

Chapter 1

Dealing with Diabetes

*1*f you've picked up this book, chances are you or someone you know has been diagnosed with diabetes. A diagnosis of any medical condition is simply a way of understanding that condition by putting it in a category that helps to predict what is likely to happen to you. A diagnosis also allows doctors and health care professionals to make assumptions about your treatment and prognosis. A diagnosis is, where possible, based on evidence.

However, if you have diabetes, you are more than a diagnosis or a measurement of abnormal blood glucose levels. You have feelings and a history. The way that you respond to the challenges of diabetes helps to determine whether the disease will be a moderate annoyance or a source of major sickness.

Also, your diabetes doesn't affect just one person. Your family, friends and colleagues are affected by how you deal with your diabetes and by their desire to help you. In this chapter, we introduce you to what it means to be diagnosed with type 1 or type 2 diabetes, the kinds of feelings you may struggle with after diagnosis and how you can move forward and learn to live with diabetes.

You Are Not Alone

Diabetes is a common disease, and getting commoner. The list of people with diabetes is long, and you may be surprised at some of the people who have it. Famous Australians like renovating expert and television personality

Rob Palmer, singer Marcia Hines, model and entrepreneur Maggie Tabberer, Olympian Dawn Fraser, ex-footballer Steve Renouf, racing car driver Jack Perkins, politician Guy Barnett and judge Barbara Holborrow have not let diabetes slow them down. Our point is that every one of these people lives with this chronic illness, and every one of them has been able to do something special with his or her life.

The names in the preceding paragraph are just a partial list of those with diabetes who are well known. The point of these examples is this: *Diabetes shouldn't stop you from doing what you want to do with your life.* We encourage you to follow the guidelines of good diabetes care, which we describe in Part III. If you follow these guidelines, you may actually be healthier than people without diabetes who smoke, overeat, underexercise, or combine these and other unhealthy habits. If you follow the guidelines of good diabetes care, you can often be just as healthy as the person without diabetes.

Living with Diabetes

Diabetes is a chronic disease that can create short- and long-term complications (see Chapters 6 and 7 for more on these complications). In some ways, dealing with a diagnosis of type 1 diabetes is quite different to dealing with a diagnosis of type 2 diabetes, and we discuss the considerations specific to each in the following sections.

Some tips for learning to live with having diabetes are common to both types, however, as follows:

- **Make sure you have good information.** Reading this book is a great start! Your next step is to find out about other reliable sources of information and support. There are excellent resources available and your diabetes care team is available to assist. Chapter 21 provides some tips to help you work out whether information available online can be trusted and Chapter 24 provides details of useful websites for further information about diabetes.

- **Get to know the doctors, nurses and other health professionals involved in your care.** Identify people you feel comfortable with and agree with on what works for you. You want to share a common vision and treatment plan with your doctor and treating team. Ensure you have a general practitioner you can relate to and stick with one rather than choosing to just turn up at a medical centre.

✔ **Keep a list of questions.** Have a 'shopping list' of questions for your doctor or diabetes care team. Write these down when you think of them and take them with you on your next visit.

✔ **Find out if you can talk to people who have managed their diabetes well.** Most people know someone with diabetes, but that doesn't mean they know what's best for you to do, or anything about your diabetes. Your diabetes care team, the Australian Diabetes Council (in NSW) or Diabetes Australia (in other states and territories) can help you get in touch with people whose circumstances are (or were) similar to yours. You may also know someone within your circle of family, friends or colleagues.

✔ **Surround yourself with loving positive support.** With luck, you not only accept the diabetes diagnosis yourself, but you also share the news with your family, friends and people close to you. Having diabetes isn't something to be ashamed of and it isn't something that you should hide from anyone. Identify who is 'there for you' and let those people know you appreciate it. If possible, give them things they can do — people do better when they have a tangible way of supporting you. See Chapter 14 for more on using the support that is available to you.

✔ **Understand how you cope with stressful situations and change and build healthy coping skills.** Diabetes often starts at times of stress — just when you don't need another thing to be happening. Being diagnosed with the condition presents you with an opportunity to reflect on how you deal with stress and what kind of coping skills you have developed. When it comes to your long-term health — both physical and mental — it pays to adopt coping skills that are healthy and help you build and maintain your motivation for making lifestyle changes. Flip over to Chapter 13 for more on healthy coping skills and motivation.

Dealing with type 1 diabetes

When you learn you have type 1 diabetes, you may become (understandably) angry that you're saddled with this 'terrible' diagnosis. Some of this anger may be at yourself, because you feel you've caused the diabetes. However, your anger only worsens your situation, including making control of your blood sugar levels more difficult. It's detrimental in the other ways too: If you target your anger at other people, they may be hurt and distance themselves from you, just when you need them. You then may also feel guilty that your anger is harming you and those close to you, which just adds more of a burden. It is important to talk this over with your diabetes care team and learn strategies for dealing with anger if you need to.

If you are feeling angry about being diagnosed with type 1 diabetes, find someone else who has had to deal with similar feelings — preferably someone who has worked through these feelings and is now managing his diabetes more positively.

Managing your type 1 diabetes may be more difficult if you:

- **Have previous mental health problems.** Talk them over with your GP or counsellor. If you have had episodes of depression, anxiety, eating disorders, substance abuse (alcohol and drugs), these can recur when you are stressed and have an effect on your diabetes.

- **Have a specific fear of needles or blood.** Get some help from a clinical psychologist — ask your GP or diabetes care team for assistance.

- **Smoke.** Start taking steps towards quitting. Ask your GP for help, call Quitline on 131 848 or go to the federal government's Quitnow website (www.quitnow.info.au).

Dealing with type 2 diabetes

Getting used to a diagnosis of diabetes can take some adjustment. Added to this, you may have an unjust stigma around type 2 diabetes. You may feel that some people think it's your fault that you developed diabetes — that it was caused simply by eating too much and not exercising enough.

As well as having to deal with the stigma attached to having type 2 diabetes, you may also have to deal with guilt. Type 2 diabetes may occur, for some, after they feel they have neglected their health. In this case, some people 'beat themselves up' after being diagnosed. While this is understandable, like anger, it is unnecessary and destructive. Think about what you can learn from your diagnosis and what steps you can take to improve your health. See Chapters 11 and 12 for more on improving your health through making changes to your diet and exercise.

If you are feeling unduly guilty about your diagnosis, you may be depressed and would benefit from talking to your doctors about it. See the section 'When you're having trouble coping' later in this chapter, and also check out Chapter 13 for more on recognising the signs of depression.

A diagnosis of type 2 diabetes may also occur in people who take certain medications (such as prednisone or olanzapine) long term. Again, developing diabetes in this case is not your fault and the medications may be something you need to continue. Talk to your doctor and diabetes care team about what medications you should be taking (and should continue to take) to ensure full physical health. Chapter 10 talks about the kinds of medications you might be prescribed for your diabetes, as well as some information on combining these drugs with drugs prescribed for other conditions.

Having type 2 diabetes can also affect, or be affected by, other aspects of your life, such as the following:

✔ **If you are overweight or unfit,** talk to your GP or specialist diabetes dietitian about developing an eating and exercise plan to improve your overall health. Some people can improve the control of their type 2 diabetes by improving their general fitness, while some cannot. Even if you still require medication to manage your diabetes, it is still worth incorporating more exercise into your daily routine, as improving fitness helps improve your general physical and mental health.

✔ **If you have previous mental health problems,** talk them over with your GP, psychologist or counsellor. If you have had episodes of depression, anxiety, eating disorders, substance abuse (alcohol, sedatives and street drugs), these can recur when you are stressed and affect your diabetes.

Diabetes is more common among people living with a mental illness. Some antipsychotic medications can lead to major weight gain, for example, while depression and anxiety can make you feel unmotivated, making it more difficult to exercise regularly and eat healthily. See Chapter 13 for more information on dealing with mental health problems common in people with diabetes.

✔ **If you have medical problems,** talk them over with your GP and diabetes care team. Your diabetes will be more stable if your general health is as good as possible.

Working On Your Mental Health

Mental health is now recognised as a key issue in the management of diabetes. People with diagnosed diabetes are twice as likely to experience depression or anxiety compared with people without diabetes. People newly diagnosed often also have to move through feelings of anger. The following sections look at these common and understandable reactions, as well as offering information on where to go for more help if your feelings of anger and depression become more long lasting.

Dealing with depression

Experts now recognise a two-way relationship exists between diabetes (types 1 and 2), stress and depression. Stress can precipitate the onset of diabetes, and ongoing diabetes-related distress has a direct effect on blood sugar levels. In turn, the pressure of living with a chronic disease can affect your mental health and capacity to cope with daily life.

Depression can make it more difficult for you to self-manage your diabetes. Depression can decrease concentration and motivation, and affect lifestyle and exercise habits, as well as pain tolerance and overall mood — which in turn affects your diabetes. If depression is not treated in people with diabetes, it can affect blood sugar levels and contribute to more diabetes-related complications.

The good news is that this cycle can be reversed. By taking steps to use more helpful ways of coping with diabetes and by treating mental illness, you can improve your mental health, increase your confidence in managing your diabetes and increase your motivation for self-care and making required lifestyle changes, such as adopting healthy eating patterns (see Chapter 11) and increasing physical activity (see Chapter 12). These changes, in turn, can improve your physical health.

Studies have clearly highlighted the kinds of coping skills, such as emotion-focused or problem-focused strategies, and the types of psychological therapies, such as motivational approaches and cognitive behavioural therapy, that are the most effective for people with diabetes. Chapter 13 goes into more detail on these types of coping styles or psychological therapies.

Getting through your anger

Anger often keeps you from successfully managing your diabetes — as long as you're angry, you're not in a problem-solving mode. Diabetes requires your focus and attention. Turn your anger into creative ways to manage your diabetes. (For ways to manage your diabetes, see Part III.)

Don't be discouraged if you're irritable, angry, guilty, anxious or miserable for a short time. These are natural coping mechanisms that serve a psychological purpose for a brief time. Allow yourself to have these feelings — and then drop them. You then need to move on and learn to live normally with your diabetes.

When you're having trouble coping

You wouldn't hesitate to seek help for your physical ailments associated with diabetes, but you may be very reluctant to seek help when you can't adjust psychologically to diabetes. The problem is that, sooner or later, your psychological problems can affect the control that you have over your diabetes. And, of course, you won't lead a very pleasant life if you're in a depressed or anxious state all the time. The following symptoms are indicators that you're past the point of handling your diabetes on your own and may be suffering from depression:

✔ You can't sleep.

✔ You have no energy when you're awake.

✔ You can't think clearly.

✔ You can't find activities that interest or amuse you.

✔ You feel worthless.

✔ You have frequent thoughts of suicide.

✔ You have no appetite.

✔ You find no humour in anything.

If you recognise several of these symptoms as features of your daily life, you need to get some help. Your sense of hopelessness may include the feeling that no-one else can help you — and that simply isn't true. Your GP, psychologist and/or endocrinologist are the people to go to for advice. They may help you to find the best treatment for your psychological difficulties.

Well-trained counsellors — especially counsellors who are trained to take care of people with diabetes — can help you find solutions that you cannot envisage in your current state. You need to find a counsellor whom you can trust so that when you're feeling low you can still talk freely, assured of the counsellor's genuine interest in your welfare.

Your doctor may decide that your situation requires medication to help treat the anxiety or depression. Currently, many drugs are available that are proven safe and relatively free of side effects. Sometimes a brief period of medication is enough to help you adjust to your diabetes.

You can also find help in a support group. The huge and continually growing number of support groups shows that positive things are happening in these groups. In most support groups, participants share their stories and problems, which helps everyone involved feel less isolated and alone.

Tips for dealing with a series of mental health issues are provided in more depth in Chapter 13.

The Way Forward After Diagnosis

You may assume that a chronic condition like diabetes will lead to a diminished quality of life for you. But must this be the case?

One factor that contributes to a lower quality of life rating is a lack of physical activity. This is a really important factor that you can alter immediately. Physical activity is a habit best maintained on a lifelong basis. The problem is that making a long-term change to a more physically active lifestyle is difficult; most people maintain their activity for a while but eventually fall back into inactive routines. See Chapter 12 for advice on exercise.

What can you do to maintain a high quality of life with diabetes? Here are the steps that accomplish the most for you:

✔ Keep your blood glucose levels as close to normal as possible (see Part III).

✔ Make exercise a regular part of your lifestyle.

✔ Get plenty of support from family, friends, and medical resources (see Chapter 14).

✔ Stay abreast of the latest developments in diabetes care (see Chapter 20).

✔ Maintain a healthy attitude.

Learning healthy ways of coping with diabetes and how to manage stress or depression can also help you cope with other challenges and improve your overall quality of life.

Chapter 2

It's the Glucose

In This Chapter

▶ Defining diabetes by the blood glucose

▶ Finding treatments for diabetes

▶ Meeting some patients and hearing their stories

The Greeks and Romans knew about diabetes. Fortunately, the way they tested for the condition — by tasting people's urine — has gone by the wayside. In this way, the Romans discovered that the urine of certain people was *mellitus,* the Latin word for *sweet.* The Greeks noticed that when people with sweet urine drank, the fluids came out in the urine almost as fast as they went in the mouth, like a siphon. They called this by the Greek word for *siphon* — *diabetes.* This is the origin of the modern name for the disease, diabetes mellitus.

In this chapter, we cover the not-so-fun stuff about diabetes — the big words, the definitions, and so on. But if you really want to understand what's happening to your body when you have diabetes, then you won't want to skip this chapter, despite the technical words.

Recognising Diabetes

The sweetness of the urine comes from *glucose,* also known as blood sugar. Many different kinds of sugars occur naturally, but glucose is the sugar that has the starring role in the body, providing a source of instant energy so that muscles can move and important chemical reactions can take place. Sugar is a carbohydrate, one group of the three sources of energy in the body. The others are protein and fat, which we discuss in greater detail in Chapter 11.

Table sugar, or *sucrose,* is actually two different kinds of sugar — glucose and fructose — linked together. Fructose is the type of sugar found in fruits and vegetables. It is sweeter than glucose, which makes sucrose sweeter than glucose as well. Your taste buds require less sucrose or fructose to get the same sweetening power of glucose.

Diabetes mellitus isn't the only condition associated with thirst and frequent urination. Another condition in which fluids go in and out of the body like a siphon is called *diabetes insipidus*. Here, the urine is not sweet. Diabetes insipidus is an entirely different disease that you shouldn't mistake for diabetes mellitus.

In order to understand the symptoms of diabetes, you need to know a little about the way the body normally handles glucose and what happens when things go wrong. The following sections cover detecting diabetes and the fine line that your body treads between control and lack of control of its glucose levels.

Testing for diabetes

The standard definition of diabetes mellitus is excessive glucose in a blood sample. For years, doctors set this level fairly high. The standard level for a normal glucose was lowered in 1997 because too many people were experiencing complications of diabetes even though they didn't have the disease by the then-current standard. The Australian standard for diagnosis endorsed by the Royal Australian College of General Practitioners (RACGP) and Diabetes Australia requires that the diagnosis of diabetes is made by using any one of the following three criteria:

- **Random plasma glucose** concentration greater than or equal to 11.1 mmol/L along with symptoms of diabetes (see the section 'Losing control of glucose' later in this chapter). The abbreviation *mmol/L* stands for *millimoles per litre*. Other countries may use the units *mg/dl*, which is *milligrams per decilitre*. To get mg/dl, you multiply mmol/L by 18.

- **Fasting plasma glucose (FPG)** of greater than or equal to 7 mmol/L. *Fasting* means that the patient has consumed no food for eight hours prior to the test.

- **Blood glucose** of greater than or equal to 11.1 mmol/L, when tested two hours (2-h PG) after ingesting 75 grams of glucose by mouth (carried out after an overnight fast following three days of adequate carbohydrate intake of greater than 200 grams per day). This test has long been known as the *oral glucose tolerance test* (OGTT). Although this test is rarely done because it takes time and is cumbersome, it remains the gold standard for the diagnosis of diabetes and should be carried out in a patient with a borderline result. This test is not necessary in patients whose random plasma glucose level is greater or equal to 11.1 mmol/L, or whose fasting plasma glucose is greater or equal to 7 mmol/L.

> If a fasting plasma glucose is between 5.5 and 7.0 mmol/L or a random plasma glucose concentration is between 7.8 mmol/L and 11.1 mmol/L on two separate occasions, an OGTT should be carried out to support or exclude a diagnosis of diabetes. If a fasting plasma glucose concentration is greater than 7 mmol/L on two separate occasions, this confirms a diagnosis of diabetes. If an OGTT is greater than 11.1 mmol/L, this confirms a diagnosis of diabetes.

Putting it another way:

- FPG less than 5.5 mmol/L is a normal fasting glucose.

- FPG greater than or equal to 6 mmol/L but less than 7.0 mmol/L is impaired fasting glucose (indicating prediabetes — see Chapter 5).

- FPG equal to or greater than 7.0 mmol/L gives a provisional diagnosis of diabetes.

During an OGTT:

- 2-h PG less than 7.8 mmol/L is normal glucose tolerance.

- 2-h PG greater than or equal to 7.8 mmol/L but less than 11.1 mmol/L is impaired glucose tolerance, which indicates disordered carbohydrate metabolism, which can lead to diabetes.

- 2-h PG equal to or greater than 11.1 mmol/L gives a diagnosis of diabetes.

Controlling glucose

A hormone called *insulin* finely controls the level of glucose in your blood. A *hormone* is a chemical substance made in one part of the body that travels (usually through the bloodstream) to a distant part of the body where it performs its work. In the case of insulin, that work is to act like a key to open the inside of a cell, such as muscle, fat or other cells, so that glucose can enter. If glucose can't enter the cell, it can provide no energy to the body.

Insulin is essential for growth. In addition to providing the key to entry of glucose into the cell, scientists consider insulin the builder hormone. It enables fat and muscle to form. It promotes storage of glucose in a form called *glycogen* for use when fuel is not coming in. It blocks breakdown of protein. Without insulin, you don't survive for long.

With this finetuning, the body manages to keep the level of glucose fairly steady at about 3.3 to 6.4 mmol/L all the time.

Losing control of glucose

Your glucose starts to rise in your blood when insulin is either not present in sufficient quantity or is not working effectively. Once your glucose rises above 10.0 mmol/L, glucose begins to spill into the urine and make it sweet. Up to that point, the kidney, the filter for the blood, is able to extract the glucose before it enters your urine. It's the loss of glucose into the urine that leads to many of the short-term complications of diabetes. (See Chapter 6 for information on short-term complications.)

The following list notes the most common early symptoms of diabetes and how they occur. One or more of the following symptoms may be present when diabetes is diagnosed:

- **Frequent urination and thirst:** The glucose in the urine draws more water out of the blood, so more urine forms. More urine in your bladder makes you feel the need to urinate more frequently during the day and to get up at night to empty the bladder, which keeps filling up. As the amount of water in your blood declines, you feel thirsty and drink much more frequently.

- **Fatigue:** Because glucose can't enter cells that depend on insulin as a key for glucose (the most important exception is the brain, which does not need insulin), glucose can't be used as a fuel to move muscles or to facilitate the many other chemical reactions that have to take place to produce energy. The person with diabetes often complains of fatigue and feels much stronger once treatment allows glucose to enter cells again.

- **Weight loss:** Weight loss is common among some people with diabetes because they lack insulin, which is the builder hormone. When insulin is lacking for any reason, the body begins to break down and you lose muscle tissue. Some of the muscle converts into glucose even though it cannot get into cells. It passes out of your body in the urine. Fat tissue breaks down into small fat particles that can provide an alternative source of energy. As your body breaks down and you lose glucose in the urine, you often experience weight loss. However, most people with diabetes are heavy rather than skinny. (We explain why in Chapter 3.)

- **Persistent vaginal infection among women:** As blood glucose rises, all the fluids in your body contain higher levels of glucose, including sweat and body secretions such as semen in men and vaginal secretions in women. Many bugs, such as bacteria and fungi, thrive in the high-glucose environment. Women begin to complain of itching or burning, an abnormal discharge from the vagina, and sometimes an odour.

Discovering Ways to Treat Diabetes

A condition that must have been diabetes mellitus appeared in the writings of China and India more than 2,000 years ago, and scholars from these two regions were the first to describe frequent urination. They also noticed the same thing that the Greeks and Romans did — urine that tasted sweet. But it wasn't until 1776 that researchers discovered the cause of the sweetness — glucose. And it wasn't until the 19th century that doctors developed a new chemical test. Later discoveries showed that the pancreas produces a crucial substance, called insulin, that controls the glucose in the blood. (For more on insulin, refer to the 'Controlling glucose' section earlier in the chapter.) Since that time, insulin has been extracted and purified enough to save many lives. Oral drugs to reduce blood glucose have become available only in the last 40 years.

Once insulin was discovered, diabetes specialists, led by Elliot Joslin and others, recommended three basic treatments for diabetes that are as valuable today as they were in 1921:

- ✔ Diet (see Chapter 11)
- ✔ Exercise (see Chapter 12)
- ✔ Medication (see Chapter 10)

The discovery of insulin didn't solve the problem of diabetes, although it immediately saved the lives of thousands of very sick individuals for whom the only 'treatment' had been starvation. As these people aged, they were found to have unexpected complications in the eyes, the kidneys and the nervous system (see Chapter 7). And insulin didn't address the problem of the much larger group of people with diabetes now known as type 2 (see Chapter 3). Their problem was not lack of insulin but resistance to its actions. Fortunately, doctors do have the tools now to bring the disease under control.

The next major discovery was the group of drugs called *sulphonylureas* (see Chapter 10), the first drugs that could be taken by mouth to lower the blood glucose. But the only way to know the level of the blood glucose was still by testing the urine, which was entirely inadequate for good control of diabetes (see Chapter 9).

Around 1980, the first portable meters for blood glucose testing became available. Now it became possible, for the first time, to relate treatment to a measurable outcome. This has led, in turn, to the discovery of other great drugs for diabetes, such as acarbose, thiazolidinediones, DPP-IV inhibitors and exanitide.

If you're not using these wonderful tools for your diabetes, you're missing the boat. You can find out exactly how to use them in Part III.

Tracking diabetes around the world

Diabetes is a global health problem. At the time of writing, an estimated 285 million people worldwide have type 2 diabetes. This figure is expected to jump to 438 million by 2030. Diabetes is concentrated where food supplies allow people to eat more kilojoules than they need so that they develop *obesity*, a condition of excessive fat. There are actually several different types of diabetes, but the type usually associated with obesity, called type 2 diabetes (see Chapter 3), far outweighs the other types.

Diabetes is also increasing throughout the world because the age of the world's population is increasing. Age is a major risk factor for diabetes along with obesity. (See Chapter 3 for more risk factors.) As other diseases are controlled and the population gets older, more diabetes is being diagnosed.

One very interesting study traces people of Japanese ancestry as they went from living in Japan to living in Hawaii and finally the United States mainland. Those in Japan, where people customarily maintain a normal weight, tended to have a very low incidence of diabetes. As they moved to Hawaii, the incidence of diabetes began to rise along with their average weight. On the US mainland, where food of all types is readily available, these Japanese had the highest rate of diabetes of all.

Not only the number of kilojoules but also the composition of the diet changes as people migrate to the United States. Before they emigrate, they tend to consume a low-fat, high-fibre diet. Once they reach their new destination, they adopt the local diet, which tends to be higher in fat and lower in fibre. The carbohydrates in the new diet are from high-energy foods, which don't tend to be filling, promoting a higher intake of kilojoules.

The Japanese provide another interesting lesson about obesity as a factor in the onset of diabetes. Japanese sumo wrestlers have to gain enormous quantities of weight in order to fight in a certain weight class. Even while they're still fighting, they demonstrate a high frequency of diabetes. Once they become more sedentary, the frequency goes up to 40 per cent, a huge prevalence.

Another group that shows the consequences of switching from a moderate kilojoule, relatively nutritious diet to a higher kilojoule diet is Aboriginal Australians. A 2004–05 study showed that the prevalence of diabetes in this group is approximately 6 per cent. However, this study had significant limitations in its methods of data collection. If prevalence rates in other indigenous groups around the world are compared to the Australian data, it becomes more likely that the prevalence of diabetes in Aboriginal Australians is between 15 and 30 per cent — or a prevalence rate between two and four times greater that for non-Aboriginal Australians.

In Australia, 7.2 per cent of the population aged between 20 and 79 years have diabetes. These numbers have doubled in the last 20 years. Currently, it is estimated that only half the people with diabetes are actually aware of it. The concern over the high incidence of diabetes led to the development of the National Diabetes Strategy (which ran from 2000 to 2004). This project was funded by more than $10 million from federal and state governments and major pharmaceutical and diagnostic companies, and its main aim was to tackle the increasing problem of diabetes and its complications in Australia. An important component of the strategy was the funding of the Australian Diabetes, Obesity and Lifestyle Study group (known as Ausdiab). This group has reported regularly on diabetes in Australia, with its most recent report being completed in 2009. Unfortunately, the strategies to improve the prevalence rates and treatment of diabetes outlined in this report have largely been ignored by governments, and no further strategic development has as yet taken place. The federal government is planning to conduct trials of an alternative model of care based mostly in the primary care sector.

Telling Typical Patient Stories

The statistics on diagnosed cases of diabetes don't begin to reflect the human dimensions of the disease. People finally take the appropriate tests after days or months (or even years) of minor discomforts that reach the point where they can no longer be tolerated. The following stories of actual patients can help you understand that diabetes is a disease that can strike people at anytime. (Please note that names have been changed.)

Jane Thomas was a 46-year-old woman who worked in a computer company and had to do a lot of standing. She noticed that she'd been having some tingling in her feet but thought it was due to all the standing. However, she had gained ten kilograms in the last six years and couldn't seem to shed them. She was beginning to wake up a few times at night to go to the bathroom. She thought this might be associated with her menopause, which was just beginning. She decided to see her local doctor, who told her everything was fine but suggested a urine analysis because she was waking up so much. To everyone's surprise, glucose was in her urine. Her doctor also did a random glucose in the lab. It was 12.5 mmol/L. He did a fasting blood glucose the next morning, and it was 9.0 mmol/L. He made a diagnosis of type 2 diabetes (see Chapter 3) and started Jane on a program of diet and exercise.

The Barlows — John, Mary, daughter, Rachel, nine, and son, Scott, five — were on a holiday to Alice Springs in December. The heat made everyone extremely thirsty and forced them to drink lots of fluids. Scott was also urinating a lot, but no-one thought much about it. However, when the family returned home, Scott continued to complain of thirst and urinated excessively. He seemed to eat a lot of sweets but didn't gain weight. Then Scott wet his bed, which hadn't happened for years. Mary felt she should take him to the paediatrician because he didn't seem like his usual active self. The doctor did a random blood glucose, which was 26 mmol/L. The doctor told Mary and John that Scott had type 1 diabetes. This was the beginning of a lot of changes in the Barlow household.

Lesley Law was a 28-year-old woman who'd just started a new job. She was eating well but losing weight. She noticed increased thirst and urination, which caused her boss to comment upon the frequent absences in the middle of work. She decided to stop drinking so many beverages, but the urination continued and she began to feel very weak. One afternoon, she fainted at the office, and an ambulance was called. At the hospital, she was found to have a blood glucose of 37.9 mmol/L. A repeat blood glucose after receiving fluids because of her very dehydrated state was 32.9 mmol/L. She was started on insulin treatment and rapidly regained her weight and her strength and returned to work after a few days.

Terry Lee was a 46-year-old black-belt taekwondo instructor. Despite his very active lifestyle, he wasn't careful about his diet and had gained seven kilograms in the last few years. He was more fatigued than he'd been in the past but blamed this on his increasing age. His mother had diabetes, but he assumed that his physical fitness would protect him from this condition. He was finding that he could barely get through a one-hour class without needing a toilet break. One of his new students had diabetes; he seemed to have more energy than Terry and never left the class during the lesson. He suggested to Terry that he ought to have the problem checked, but Terry insisted that he couldn't possibly have diabetes with all his activity. The symptoms of fatigue and frequent urination got worse, and he finally made an appointment with his GP. Blood tests revealed a random blood glucose of 14.7 mmol/L. The following week, a fasting blood glucose was done through the laboratory — 11.2 mmol/L. The doctor told Terry he had diabetes, but Terry refused to believe it. He left the doctor's office in an angry mood but vowed to lose weight and did so successfully. On a repeat visit to the doctor, a random glucose was 9.3 mmol/L. He told the doctor that he knew he didn't have diabetes. However, he continued to feel lethargic and was constantly getting up at night to go to the bathroom. He put up with these symptoms for another six weeks, but finally returned to the doctor. He was again found to have a random blood glucose of 16.8 mmol/L. Finally, he accepted the diagnosis and started treatment. He rapidly returned to his usual state of health, and the fatigue disappeared. He was a bit cross with himself for being so stubborn!

Debbie Miller's active sex life with her husband was continually being interrupted by vaginal yeast infections, which resulted in an unpleasant odour, redness and itching. She would go to the chemist and purchase an over-the-counter preparation, which promptly cured the condition but it rapidly returned. Finally, after three of these infections in two months, she was advised by the pharmacist to see her local doctor for further testing. Her doctor ordered a variety of tests including a fasting blood glucose, which was 8.3 mmol/L. The doctor told her she had diabetes and recommended exercise and diet to start with. Exercise and diet not only lowered her blood glucose to the point that she no longer developed yeast infections, but also resulted in weight loss and return of energy that made her sex life with her husband even more satisfying.

Chapter 3

What Type of Diabetes Do You Have?

. . . .

. . . .

The information in this chapter should put you on closer terms with your pancreas, which is good, because you need your pancreas just as much as it needs you. Most of the time, your pancreas hides behind your stomach quietly doing its work, helping with digestion first and then helping to make use of the digested food. In one way or another, the pancreas plays a role in all of the various types of diabetes.

In this chapter, we explain how you identify whether you're at risk of type 1 or type 2 diabetes and how they are acquired. We also cover the causes of diabetes. (You can find information on how both types of diabetes may be prevented in Chapter 4.)

This chapter also helps you get a clear understanding of your type of diabetes, how it relates to the other types of diabetes, and how the failure of your pancreas to do its assigned job can lead to a number of unfortunate consequences (covered in greater detail in Part II).

Getting to Know Your Pancreas

The pancreas has two major functions. One is to produce *digestive enzymes*, which are the chemicals in your small intestine that help to break down the food that you eat. The digestive enzymes don't have much relation to diabetes, so we won't focus on them in this book. Your pancreas's other function is to produce and secrete directly into the blood a hormone of major importance: *Insulin*.

Figure 3-1 shows the cellular make-up of the pancreas. The cells that are relevant to diabetes are the beta cells, which produce the key hormone, insulin, and the alpha cells, which produce glucagon, a hormone that raises glucose levels. The insulin-producing pancreas cells are found in groups called *Islets of Langerhans*.

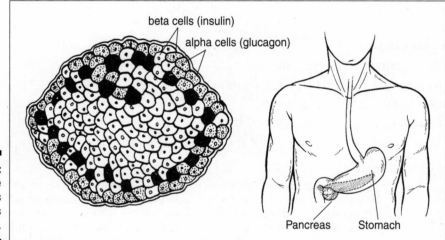

beta cells (insulin)

alpha cells (glucagon)

Pancreas   Stomach

Figure 3-1:
The pancreas and its parts.

If you understand only one hormone in your body, insulin should be that hormone (especially if you want to understand diabetes). Over the course of your life, the insulin that your body produces or the insulin that you inject into your body (see Chapter 10) affects whether or not you control your diabetes and avoid the complications of the disease.

Think of your insulin as an insurance agent, who lives in Sydney (which is your pancreas) but travels from there to do business in Melbourne (your muscles), Brisbane (your fat tissue), Adelaide (your liver), and other places. This insulin insurance agent is insuring your good health.

Wherever insulin travels in your body, it opens up the cells so that glucose can enter them. After it enters them, the cells can immediately use glucose for energy, store it in a storage form of glucose (called *glycogen*) for rapid use later on, or convert it to fat for use even later as energy.

After glucose leaves your blood and enters your cells, your blood glucose level falls. Your pancreas can detect when your glucose level is falling, and it turns off the release of insulin to prevent unhealthy low levels of blood glucose called *hypoglycaemia* from developing (see Chapter 6). At the same time, your liver begins to release glucose from storage and makes new glucose from amino acids in your blood.

If your insurance agent (insulin) doesn't show up when you need him (meaning that you have an absence of insulin, as in type 1 diabetes) or he does a poor job when he does show up (such as when you have a resistance to insulin, as in type 2 diabetes), your insurance coverage may be very poor (in which case, your blood glucose starts to climb). High blood glucose is where all your problems begin.

Medical research has proved conclusively that high blood glucose is bad for the body, and that keeping the levels of blood glucose as normal as possible prevents the complications of diabetes (see Part II). Most treatments for diabetes are directed at restoring the blood glucose to normal.

You Have Type 1 Diabetes

John Phillips, a six-year-old boy, was always very active, and his parents became concerned when his teacher told them that John didn't seem to have much energy during a school camp. When he got home from the camp, John's parents noticed that he seemed to be thirsty all the time and was always running to the toilet. Although John was very hungry and was eating more than enough, he seemed to be losing weight. His parents took him to a paediatrician, who did several blood glucose tests and told them that their son was suffering from type 1 diabetes mellitus, a condition which used to be called *insulin-dependent diabetes mellitus* (IDDM) or *juvenile onset diabetes*.

This story has a happy ending because John's parents, although very upset at this discovery, were willing to do everything necessary to bring John's glucose under control. These days, John is as energetic as ever, but he has had to get used to a few inconveniences in his daily routine. (We cover such daily lifestyle changes in Part III.)

In the following sections, we describe the symptoms and causes of type 1 diabetes, and how likely it is that you may suffer from it.

Identifying the symptoms of type 1 diabetes

Before your doctor actually diagnoses diabetes, you may notice — in yourself or your child — some of the major signs and symptoms of type 1 diabetes. If you experience the following symptoms, ask your doctor whether it is possible that you have diabetes:

- ✔ **Frequent urination:** You experience frequent urination because your kidneys can't return all the glucose to your bloodstream when your blood glucose level is greater than 10 mmol/L. (See Chapter 9 for details on blood glucose level testing.) The large amount of glucose in your urine makes the urine so concentrated that water is drawn out of the blood and into the urine to reduce the concentration of glucose in the urine. This water and glucose fill up the bladder repeatedly.

- ✔ **Increased thirst:** Your thirst increases as you experience frequent urination, because you lose so much water in the urine that your body begins to dehydrate.

- ✔ **Increased hunger:** You notice that you're increasingly hungry. Your body has plenty of extra glucose in the blood, but your hunger is a result of your cells becoming malnourished because you lack insulin to allow the glucose to enter into your cells. Your body is going through 'hunger in the midst of plenty'.

- ✔ **Weight loss:** You lose weight as your body loses glucose in the urine and your body breaks down muscle and fat looking for energy.

- ✔ **Weakness:** You feel weak and tired because your muscle cells and other tissues don't get the energy that they require from glucose.

Type 1 diabetes used to be called *juvenile onset diabetes* because it occurred most frequently in children. However, so many cases are now found in adults that doctors don't use the term 'juvenile' anymore. Some children are diagnosed early in life, and other children experience the onset of the disease as they get a little older.

With older children, the early signs and symptoms of diabetes may have been missed by parents, sports coaches or teachers. These children have a great deal of fat breakdown in their bodies to provide energy, and this fat breakdown creates other problems. *Ketones*, products of the breakdown of fats, begin to accumulate in the blood and spill into the urine. Ketones are acidic and lead to nausea, abdominal pain and sometimes vomiting.

At the same time as the fat is breaking down, the child's blood glucose rises higher. Levels as high as 22.2 to 33.3 mmol/L are not uncommon, but levels as low as 16.6 mmol/L are possible. The child's blood is like syrup and doesn't circulate as freely as normal. The large amount of water leaving the body with the glucose depletes important substances such as sodium and potassium. The vomiting causes the child to lose more fluids and body substances. All these abnormalities cause the child to become very drowsy and possibly lose consciousness. This situation is called *diabetic ketoacidosis*, and if it isn't identified and corrected soon, the child may not survive. (See Chapter 6 for details on the symptoms, causes and treatments of ketoacidosis.)

A few special circumstances affect the symptoms that you may see in people with type 1 diabetes. Remember the following factors:

- ✔ **The 'honeymoon' period** is a time after the diagnosis of diabetes, when the person's insulin needs decline for one to six months and the disease seems to get milder. The honeymoon period is longer when a child is older at the time of diagnosis, but the apparent diminishing of the disease is always temporary.

- ✔ **Males and females** get type 1 diabetes to an equal degree.

- ✔ **Warm summer months** are associated with a decrease in the occurrence of diabetes compared to the winter months, particularly in older children. The probable reason for this is that a virus is involved in bringing on diabetes, and viruses spread much more when children are learning and playing together inside in the winter.

Investigating the causes of type 1 diabetes

When your doctor diagnoses you with type 1 diabetes, you almost immediately begin to wonder what could have caused you to acquire the disease. Did someone with diabetes sneeze on you? Did you eat so much sugary food that your body reacted by giving you diabetes? Well, rest assured that the causes of diabetes aren't so simple or easily avoidable.

Type 1 diabetes is an *autoimmune disease*, meaning that your body is unkind enough to react against — and, in this case, destroy — a vital part of itself, namely the insulin-producing beta cells of the pancreas. One way that doctors discovered that type 1 diabetes is an autoimmune disease was by measuring proteins in the blood, called *antibodies*, which are literally substances directed against your body — and, in particular, against your islet cells. These antibodies are called *islet cell antibodies*.

In type 1 diabetes, a specific antibody called the *glutamic acid decarboxylase (GAD) antibody* is often present. The detection of GAD antibodies is useful to distinguish between type 1 and type 2 diabetes. The GAD antibodies can be found in some relatives of people who have type 1 diabetes and in people a few years before they develop diabetes. However, the incidence of type 1 diabetes is sporadic and in 90 per cent of cases the person will have no relatives with type 1 diabetes.

Another clue that type 1 diabetes is an autoimmune disease is that treatments to reduce autoimmunity also delay the onset of type 1 diabetes. Also, type 1 diabetes tends to occur in people who have other known autoimmune diseases.

Knowledge of genetic markers may be helpful in assessing the risk of type 1 diabetes developing in close relatives of a person with type 1 diabetes. Several genes are involved but the major ones are in the Human Leucocyte Antigen (HLA) region of the chromosomes. Use of these genetic markers, in addition to antibody levels in the blood and a family history of diabetes, make it possible to estimate the risk of developing type 1 diabetes. However, because 90 per cent of people don't have a family history of type 1 diabetes, DNA screening is not a clinically useful routine diagnostic tool, and in Australia it is usually only used for research purposes.

The presence of certain genetic markers on your chromosomes isn't enough to guarantee that you'll get diabetes. Many people who have these characteristics never get diabetes, so doctors need to consider other factors in addition to your DNA.

Another essential factor in predicting whether you will develop diabetes is your exposure to something in the environment, most likely a virus. If this virus infiltrates your body, it can cause diabetes by attacking your pancreas directly and diminishing your ability to produce insulin, which quickly creates the diabetic condition in your body. The virus can also cause diabetes if it's made up of a substance that's also naturally present in your pancreas. If the virus and your pancreas possess the same substance, the antibodies that your body produces to fight off the virus will also attack the shared substance in your pancreas, leaving you in the same condition as if the virus itself attacked your pancreas.

Researchers haven't identified one particular virus that they can blame for type 1 diabetes. Research on people who are at the beginning stages of type 1 diabetes has uncovered many different viruses that could be the culprit (including rubella infection during pregnancy). The type 1 diabetes virus may be the same as a virus that causes the common cold.

Getting type 1 diabetes

You may get type 1 diabetes if you have certain factors on your *chromosomes*, the DNA in each cell in your body that determines your physical characteristics. If you have several of these factors, your chance of getting type 1 diabetes is much greater than that of a person who has none of these factors.

But just having these factors is not usually enough. You have to come in contact with something in your environment that triggers the destruction of your *beta cells*, the cells that make insulin. Doctors think that this environmental trigger is probably a virus, and they've identified several viruses that may be to blame (see preceding section). People with type 1 diabetes probably get the virus just like any cold virus — from someone who has the virus who sneezes on them. But because they also have the genetic tendency, they get type 1 diabetes.

A small number of people with type 1 diabetes don't seem to need an environmental factor to trigger the diabetes. In them, the disease is entirely an autoimmune destruction of the beta cells. If you fall into this category of people with diabetes, you may have other autoimmune diseases such as autoimmune thyroid disease.

How likely are you to get type 1 diabetes if your brother or sister gets it? Studies of many families have provided fairly good answers to this question. If one of your parents has type 1 diabetes, the odds are only about 6 per cent that you will get it (it's a higher risk if your father has type 1 diabetes than if your mother does). You get half of your total genetic material from each parent.

The identical twin of a person with type 1 diabetes has about a 30 to 40 per cent chance of also getting type 1 diabetes. If you have only half of your genetic material in common with your sibling who has type 1 diabetes, your chance of getting type 1 diabetes drops to 5 per cent. If none of the genetic material associated with diabetes is the same as your sibling with type 1 diabetes, your chance of developing type 1 diabetes is less than 2 per cent.

The relatively low chances of both siblings — even for identical twins — getting diabetes clearly show that more factors than your genetic inheritance from your parents are involved in acquiring type 1 diabetes. If this weren't the case, identical twins would both have type 1 diabetes almost 100 per cent of the time.

You Have Type 2 Diabetes

Rosemary Stevens, a 46-year-old woman who is 1.65 metres tall, found she weighed about 70 kilograms, which meant she had gained about 5 kilograms over a year. Rosemary had noticed that she felt more tired than usual, even though she didn't do much exercise. However, she blamed her busy lifestyle and recent weight gain for her fatigue. Another reason for Rosemary feeling more tired was that she had to get up several times a night to urinate, which was unusual for her.

Rosemary was especially disturbed because her vision had become blurry, and she did a lot of computer work. She finally went to see her GP when she developed a rash and discharge from her vagina. When Rosemary described her symptoms, her GP diagnosed thrush and decided to do a blood glucose test. Rosemary's blood glucose level that afternoon registered at 12.2 mmol/L.

Rosemary's GP asked her whether members of her family had diabetes, and she replied that her mother and a sister were both being treated for it. The doctor also asked Rosemary about any tingling in her feet, and she admitted that she had noticed some tingling for the past few months but didn't think it was important. Then her GP ordered a fasting blood glucose test from the laboratory, it came back at 9.4 mmol/L. Rosemary's GP had to tell her that she had type 2 diabetes. Her cholesterol and trigylcerides (blood fats) were also outside the recommended range. Rosemary's GP then checked her blood pressure, which was also elevated. Her GP then explained to her that these problems — diabetes, high blood fats and a high blood pressure — were linked and were often diagnosed at the same time.

The signs and symptoms that Rosemary manifested, along with the results of the two blood glucose tests, provide a textbook picture of type 2 diabetes. (Type 2 diabetes used to be known as *non–insulin dependent diabetes mellitus* (NIDDM) or *maturity onset diabetes*.) However, people with type 2 diabetes may have few or none of these symptoms. That is why it is so important for your doctor to check your blood glucose level on a regular basis. (We discuss how often you should do this test in Chapter 9.)

Type 2 diabetes typically begins around the age of 40 and increases in frequency as you get older. However, its incidence is becoming more frequent in young children and younger adults. Because the symptoms are so mild at first, you may not notice them. You may ignore these symptoms for years before they become bothersome enough to consult your doctor. So type 2 diabetes is a disease of gradual onset rather than the severe emergency that can herald type 1 diabetes. No autoimmunity is involved in type 2 diabetes, so no antibodies are found. Doctors believe that no virus is involved in the onset of type 2 diabetes.

Recent statistics show that, throughout the world, ten times more people have type 2 diabetes than type 1. Part II tells you about the possible complications of diabetes, and Part III covers treatments that can help you prevent these complications.

Identifying the symptoms of type 2 diabetes

A fairly large percentage of the population of Australia (approximately 1.1 million people, which is equivalent to 85 per cent of all cases of diabetes) has type 2 diabetes. The following signs and symptoms are good indicators that you have type 2 diabetes. If you experience two or more of these symptoms, check with your doctor:

- **Fatigue:** Type 2 diabetes makes you tired because your body's cells aren't getting the glucose fuel that they need. Even though there's plenty of insulin, your body is resistant to its actions. (Refer to the earlier section 'Getting to Know Your Pancreas' for further explanation.)

- **Frequent urination and thirst:** You find yourself urinating more frequently than usual, which dehydrates your body and leaves you thirsty.

- **Blurred vision:** The lenses of your eyes swell and shrink as your blood glucose levels rise and fall. Your vision blurs because your eyes can't adjust quickly enough to these changes in the lenses.

- **Slow healing of skin, gum and urinary infections:** Your white blood cells, which help with healing and defend your body against infections, don't function correctly in the high-glucose environment of your body when it has diabetes. Unfortunately, the bugs that cause infections thrive in the same high-glucose environment, so diabetes leaves your body especially susceptible to infections.

- **Genital itching:** Yeast infections also love a high-glucose environment. So diabetes is often accompanied by the itching and discomfort of yeast infections.

- **Numbness in the feet or legs:** You experience numbness because of a common long-term complication of diabetes, called *neuropathy*. (We explain neuropathy in Chapter 7.) If you notice numbness along with the other symptoms of diabetes, you probably have had the disease for quite a while, because neuropathy takes more than five years to develop in a person with diabetes.

✔ **Heart disease:** Heart disease occurs much more often in people with type 2 diabetes than in the non-diabetic population. However, heart disease may appear when you are merely *glucose-intolerant* (which we explain in the next section), before you actually have diagnosable diabetes.

✔ **Obesity:** If you're obese, you are considerably more likely to acquire diabetes than you would be if you maintained your ideal weight. (See Chapter 11 to find out how to calculate your target weight.) Not all obese people develop diabetes, however, so obesity isn't a definite indication of diabetes.

In some cases, the signs and symptoms of type 2 diabetes (such as high blood glucose) are similar to the symptoms of type 1 diabetes (refer to the section 'Identifying the symptoms of type 1 diabetes' earlier in this chapter). In many ways, though, the two types differ. The following points set out some of the differences between symptoms in type 1 and type 2 diabetes:

✔ **Age of onset:** Those with type 1 diabetes are usually younger than those with type 2 diabetes.

✔ **Body weight:** Those with type 1 diabetes are thin or normal in weight, while obesity is a common characteristic of those with type 2 diabetes.

✔ **Level of glucose:** Those with type 1 diabetes have higher glucose levels at the onset of the disease.

✔ **Severity of onset:** Type 1 diabetes usually has a much more severe onset, while type 2 diabetes gradually shows its symptoms.

Investigating the causes of type 2 diabetes

Although type 2 diabetes doesn't usually appear in your body until later in life (as opposed to the early onset of type 1 diabetes), if you've been diagnosed with type 2 diabetes, you're probably nonetheless shocked and curious about why you developed the disease. Doctors have learnt quite a bit about the causes of type 2 diabetes. For example, they know that type 2 diabetes runs in families. Usually, people with type 2 diabetes can find a relative who has had the disease. Therefore, doctors consider type 2 diabetes to be much more of a genetic disease than type 1 diabetes.

In studies of identical twins, when one twin has type 2 diabetes, the likelihood that type 2 diabetes will develop in the other twin is between 75 and 90 per cent. A number of ongoing studies are investigating the susceptibility genes associated with the development of type 2 diabetes. However, it is known that the genes associated with type 2 diabetes aren't the same as those associated with type 1.

Developing insulin resistance

People with type 2 diabetes have plenty of insulin in their bodies (unlike people with type 1 diabetes, who have none of their own insulin in their bodies), but their bodies respond to the insulin in abnormal ways. Those with type 2 diabetes are *insulin-resistant*, meaning that their bodies resist the normal, healthy functioning of insulin. This insulin resistance, combined with not producing enough insulin to overcome the insulin resistance, causes type 2 diabetes, just like the absent insulin causes type 1 diabetes.

Even before obesity sets in, or the person does no exercise, or diabetes is present, future type 2 patients already show signs of insulin resistance. First of all, the level of insulin in the blood of these people is elevated compared to the level found in normal people. Secondly, an injection of insulin doesn't reduce the blood glucose in these insulin-resistant people nearly as much as it does in people without insulin resistance. (See Chapter 10 for more about insulin injections in diabetes.)

When your body needs to make extra insulin just to keep your blood glucose normal, your insulin is, obviously, less effective than it should be — which means that you have *impaired glucose tolerance* or *prediabetes* (see Chapter 5). Your body goes through impaired glucose tolerance before you actually have diabetes, because your blood glucose is still lower than the levels needed for a diagnosis of diabetes (refer to Chapter 2). When you have impaired glucose tolerance and you add other factors such as weight gain, a sedentary lifestyle or ageing, your pancreas can't keep up with your insulin demands and you develop diabetes.

Another factor that comes into play when doctors make a diagnosis of type 2 diabetes is the release of sugar from your liver, known as your *hepatic glucose output*. Why is your glucose high in the morning after you've fasted all night if you have type 2 diabetes? You would think that your glucose would be low because you haven't eaten any sugar that would increase your body's glucose. In fact, your liver is a storage bank for a lot of glucose, and it can make even more from other substances in the body. As your insulin resistance increases, your liver begins to release glucose inappropriately and your fasting blood glucose rises.

Dispelling myths about the causes of type 2 diabetes

People often think that the following factors cause type 2 diabetes, but they actually have nothing to do with the onset of the disease:

- ✔ **Antibodies:** Antibodies against islet cells are not a major factor in type 2 diabetes. Type 2 diabetes isn't an autoimmune disease like type 1.

- ✔ **Diabetic ketoacidosis:** Type 2 diabetes isn't generally associated with diabetic ketoacidosis (see Chapter 6). People with type 2 diabetes are ketosis-resistant, except under extremely severe stress caused by infections or trauma. (Also refer to Chapter 6 for a discussion of *hyperglycaemic hyperosmolar state*, a related condition in which people with type 2 diabetes have extremely high glucose but don't have the fat breakdown that leads to ketoacidosis.)

- ✔ **Emotions:** Changes in your emotions don't play a large role in the development of type 2 diabetes, but may be very important in dealing with diabetes mellitus and subsequent control.

- ✔ **Gender:** Males and females are equally as likely to develop type 2 diabetes. Gender doesn't play a role in the onset of this disease.

- ✔ **Stress:** Too much stress isn't a major cause of diabetes.

- ✔ **Sugar:** Eating excessive amounts of sugar doesn't cause diabetes — although it may bring out the disease to the extent that it makes you fat. Eating too much protein or fat will do the same thing.

Getting type 2 diabetes

Genetic inheritance causes type 2 diabetes. However, lifestyle factors such as obesity and lack of exercise interact with genetic risk to trigger the disease. People with type 2 diabetes are insulin-resistant before they become obese or sedentary or undergo surgery. Subsequently, ageing, poor eating habits, obesity and failure to exercise combine to bring out the disease.

Inheritance seems to be a much stronger factor in type 2 diabetes than in type 1 diabetes. The chance that a parent with type 2 diabetes will have a child with type 2 diabetes (assuming that the other parent doesn't have the disease) is about 10 per cent. An identical twin of a person with type 2 diabetes is at high risk — between 75 per cent and 90 per cent — of getting the disease. If you are the non-identical brother or sister of someone with type 2 diabetes, you also have a strong chance of developing it. These are much higher figures than for type 1 diabetes.

Women with *polycystic ovary disease* are another high-risk group. Polycystic ovary disease is a common condition in women who have an over-secretion of insulin causing irregular menstrual cycles, facial hair and acne.

A number of early warning signs appear in populations that are most at risk of developing type 2 diabetes. In developing countries, where often people do not have enough food, those whose genetic makeup enables their bodies to use carbohydrates in a very efficient manner have an advantage over the rest of the population because they can survive on a low intake of food and kilojoules. Perhaps when they were young, these people didn't make enough insulin-producing cells because they didn't need them for their reduced food intake. If these people then receive ample supplies of food, their bodies are overwhelmed. Their pancreases may not have enough insulin-producing cells to handle the load and they're likely to become fat and sedentary and develop diabetes. This may explain why people in developing countries are the most at risk of developing type 2 diabetes. Population studies show that the incidence of diabetes is greatest in developing countries such as China and India.

You Have Gestational Diabetes

If you're pregnant and you've never had diabetes, it's possible that during the course of your pregnancy you could acquire a form of diabetes called *gestational diabetes*. Gestational diabetes occurs in about 5 per cent of all pregnancies.

While you're pregnant, the growing foetus and the placenta create various hormones to help the foetus to grow and develop properly. Some of these hormones have other characteristics, such as anti-insulin properties, that decrease your body's sensitivity to insulin, increase glucose production, and therefore cause diabetes.

At approximately your 20th week of pregnancy, your body produces enough of these hormones to block your insulin's normal actions and cause diabetes. After you give birth, the foetus and placenta are no longer in your body, so their anti-insulin hormones are gone and your diabetes disappears in most cases.

Be aware that, even though your diabetes subsides after you give birth, type 2 diabetes develops within 5 to 15 years after the pregnancy in 10 to 50 per cent of women who have had gestational diabetes. This high risk of type 2 diabetes probably results from a genetic susceptibility to diabetes in certain women, a susceptibility that is magnified by the large amount of anti-insulin hormones in their bodies during pregnancy.

Your obstetrician or midwife may require you to do a screening test for gestational diabetes between the 26th and 28th week of your pregnancy. This test is done by taking a sample of blood to check its glucose level. An hour later, the test is repeated after you have consumed a very sweet drink. If this screening test is abnormal, you will be sent along for a two-hour oral glucose tolerance test (OGTT) to see if you have gestational diabetes. (See Chapter 18 for more on doing an OGTT, and for more discussion of pregnancy and diabetes.)

Could You Have Another Type of Diabetes?

Cases of diabetes other than type 1, type 2 or gestational are rare and usually don't cause severe symptoms in the people who have them. But occasionally one of these rare types of diabetes is responsible for a severe case of the disease. The following outlines the symptoms and causes of other types of diabetes:

- ✔ **Diabetes due to loss or disease of pancreatic tissue:** If you have a disease such as cancer that necessitates the removal of some of your pancreas, you lose your pancreas's valuable insulin-producing beta cells and your body becomes diabetic. This form of diabetes isn't always severe because you lose *glucagon*, another hormone found in your pancreas, after pancreatic surgery. Glucagon blocks insulin action in your body, so when your body has less glucagon, it can function with less insulin, leaving you with a milder case of diabetes.

- ✔ **Diabetes due to chronic pancreatitis:** Diabetes can also develop in people who have *chronic pancreatitis* (inflammation of the pancreas) due to excessive alcohol consumption.

- ✔ **Diabetes due to other diseases:** Your body has a number of hormones that block insulin action or have actions that are opposed to insulin's actions. You produce these hormones in glands other than your pancreas. If you get a tumour on one of these hormone-producing

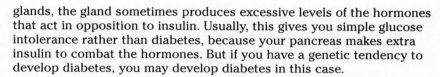

glands, the gland sometimes produces excessive levels of the hormones that act in opposition to insulin. Usually, this gives you simple glucose intolerance rather than diabetes, because your pancreas makes extra insulin to combat the hormones. But if you have a genetic tendency to develop diabetes, you may develop diabetes in this case.

✔ **Diabetes due to hormone treatments for other diseases:** If you're receiving hormones to treat a disease other than diabetes, those hormones could cause diabetes in your body. The hormone that is most likely to cause diabetes in this situation is *hydrocortisone* (similar drugs are prednisone and dexamethasone), an anti-inflammatory agent used in diseases of inflammation (such as arthritis). If you're taking hydrocortisone and you have the symptoms of diabetes listed in earlier sections of this chapter, talk to your doctor.

✔ **Diabetes due to other drugs:** If you're taking other commonly used drugs, be aware that some of them raise your blood glucose as a side effect. Some antihypertensive drugs, especially *hydrochlorothiazide*, raise your blood glucose level. *Nicotinic acid*, a drug occasionally used for lowering cholesterol, also raises your blood glucose. If you have a genetic tendency towards diabetes, taking these drugs may be enough to give you the disease.

✔ **Diabetes due directly to genetic inheritance:** Both type 1 and, particularly, type 2 diabetes are caused by a combination of genetic and environmental risk factors. However, other forms of diabetes are directly inherited due to one abnormal gene. These genetics are very rare but, if you have a family history of one of these types of disorders or your endocrinologist suspects you may have one of these rare conditions, you may be asked if you wish to have genetic testing. This testing is currently not performed in Australia and the tests have to be sent overseas. While in some cases this is free, in other cases a fee will be charged.

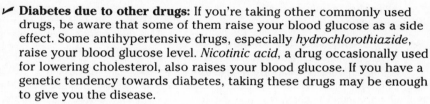

Conditions and hormones that can lead to diabetes

The following is a partial list of hormones caused by tumours and their associated conditions:

✔ Excessive adrenal gland hormone (cortisol) is present in *Cushing's Syndrome*. *Cortisol* stimulates the liver to produce more glucose while it blocks the uptake of glucose by muscle tissue.

✔ Excessive growth hormone is made by a tumour of the pituitary gland resulting in *acromegaly*. Growth hormone reduces insulin sensitivity and forces the pancreas to make much more insulin.

(continued)

(continued)

- Excessive adrenaline is made by a *phaeochromocytoma* (a tumour of another part of the adrenal gland). It causes increased liver production of glucose, while it blocks insulin secretion.

- Excessive aldosterone is made by still another part of the adrenal gland in a condition called *primary hyperaldosteronism* or Conn's syndrome. This condition causes glucose intolerance in a different way — by facilitating the loss of body potassium, which has a negative effect on insulin production.

- Excessive thyroid hormone found in *hyperthyroidism* causes the liver and other organs to produce excessive quantities of glucose. Hyperthyroidism is also a disease of autoimmunity, which may play a role in the loss of glucose tolerance.

- A *glucagon secreting tumour of the pancreas* can create excessive glucagon. Glucagon has many properties that are opposite to insulin. This condition is rare, and only around 100 cases of it have been described in medical literature, so don't think you have it.

- A *somatostatin secreting tumour of the pancreas* can create excessive somatostatin. Somatostatin is another hormone made in a cell present in the Islets of Langerhans. Somatostatin actually blocks insulin from leaving the beta cell, but it also blocks glucagon and other hormones, so the diabetes is very mild. This condition occurs even less often than the glucagon secreting tumour.

- Excessive prolactin is present in a *prolactin secreting tumour of the pituitary gland*. It blocks insulin action and glucose intolerance results.

Chapter 4

Taking Preventive Measures

*Y*ou can prevent diabetes, but not quite as easily as you may like. While the best way of ensuring you never suffer from diabetes is to pick your parents carefully, that's a little bit impractical, even with modern technology.

In general, you can prevent a disease if it meets two requirements. Firstly, you have to be able to identify individuals who are at high risk of getting the disease. Secondly, the disease must have at least some treatments or actions that you can take to definitely reduce the onset of the disease.

In this chapter, we cover how you can fulfil each of these requirements in the effort to prevent the occurrence of both type 1 and type 2 diabetes.

We also outline the negative effects that diabetes has not only on a person suffering from diabetes but on the entire medical system in Australia, and also discuss research and programs in the field of prevention. First, though, we demonstrate graphically to what extent diabetes is on the increase.

Getting to Grips with the Rise in Diabetes

So that you can appreciate just why it's so important to prevent diabetes, the following two charts illustrate the upward trend in diabetes in Australia. The first chart, Figure 4-1, shows the rate of diabetes across Australia in 2001; Figure 4-2 shows the rate in 2004 to 2005. The data used to create these charts comes from two different sources — the National Health Survey and the National Diabetes Services Scheme — but the results are almost identical. (The NHS data includes those with gestational diabetes while the NDSS data doesn't.)

As the two charts show, a pattern of increasing prevalence with increasing age is evident in Australia.

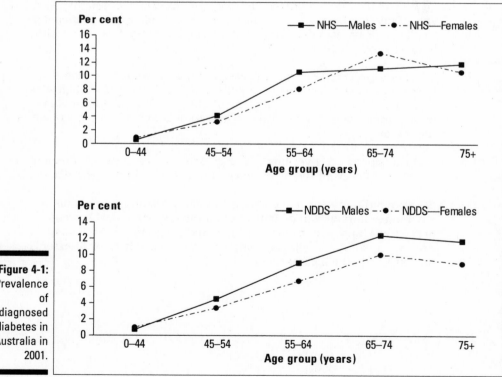

Figure 4-1:
Prevalence
of
diagnosed
diabetes in
Australia in
2001.

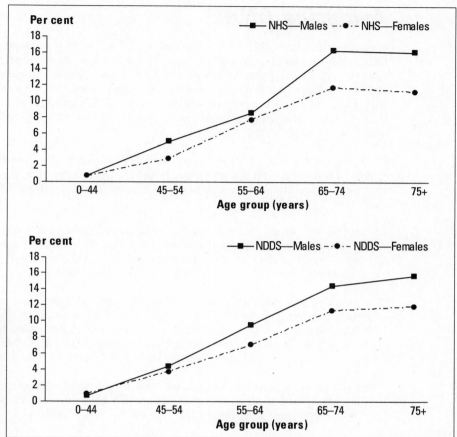

Figure 4-2: Prevalence of diagnosed diabetes in Australia in 2004–05.

Counteracting Type 1 Diabetes

Medical science is undertaking research in a range of areas that may be able to provide information on what factors influence or can even predict the onset of type 1 diabetes. Current research focuses on gene research and immunological interventions. Extensive research trials have also been conducted to try to prevent the destruction of the beta cells, the cells in the pancreas that make the vital hormone insulin (refer to Chapter 3 for more information).

Analysing DNA

You may think that all the recent scientific advances in gene research would enable doctors to change people's genetic material in order to prevent the onset of type 1 diabetes. Although scientists have certainly made great strides in identifying the genes associated with susceptibility to diabetes, they haven't reached the point where they can safely change those genes. Unfortunately, the prevention of type 1 diabetes through gene manipulation won't be possible for a long time yet.

For the moment, though, research scientists can analyse the genetic material (DNA) of a person with a family history of type 1 diabetes to see whether that person has the genetic material most often found in people who have diabetes.

At the time of writing, several studies in Australia and overseas are looking at the development of type 1 diabetes in individuals, with the hope that gaining a better understanding of the progression of diabetes will help to eventually prevent diabetes or provide a cure in the future.

The result of this analysis, together with islet cell, GAD and insulin antibody profiles, can be used to make a prediction of whether the person will develop diabetes (refer to Chapter 3). If the risk is estimated to be high, they may be eligible to enter a diabetes prevention trial. (See www. diabetestrials.org for more on prevention trials running in Australia.)

Although no treatment has been found to prevent type 1 diabetes in at-risk individuals, type 1 is an excellent candidate for prevention trials because of the often long latent time before the disease becomes obvious.

Most of the prevention trials are conducted in the knowledge that people whose bodies produce autoantibodies are at risk of getting, or already have, type 1 diabetes and that the antibodies are gradually destroying their insulin-producing beta cells (refer to Chapter 3 for more information). In these people, full-blown type 1 diabetes may take a couple of years to appear and subsequently create major problems, so there may be time to intervene with one of the methods developed to counter autoimmunity.

Investigating the diets of newborn babies

Whether the early introduction of cow's milk, wheat or gluten into the diet of a newborn (that is, before three months of age) is associated with the development of type 1 diabetes remains unresolved.

A recent review of the literature relating to the clinical studies in this area concluded that no specific nutrient or dietary factor had been conclusively shown to play a role in the development of type 1 diabetes. However, sufficient questions still exist about these theories and studies are ongoing.

Vaccinating against diabetes

Another example of prevention for type 1 diabetes would be getting a vaccination against viruses associated with diabetes. Unfortunately, doctors haven't yet pinpointed the exact virus or viruses, so vaccinations aren't practical at the present time. In some countries where type 1 diabetes occurs often — for example, Finland — doctors have tried vaccinations but this didn't stop the rise in the number of new cases of type 1 diabetes.

Doctors also have considered giving antiviral agents to people who are at high risk of acquiring diabetes, but so far this approach has only been successful in animal testing.

Protecting the body's own source of insulin

The most prevalent methods of prevention for type 1 diabetes attempt to block the autoimmune disease from destroying all of the pancreas's beta cells. Some of the research trials that have been carried out involve the following:

- ✔ **Immunosuppressive drugs:** Drugs which alter the body's immune response (used nowadays following organ transplantation), such as steroids, cyclosporin and azathioprine, have been given to people just before and just after the diagnosis of type 1 diabetes to try to undo — or at least slow down — the body's destruction of pancreatic beta cells. Although studies over the last two or three decades have showed some reduction in insulin requirements in people taking these drugs as compared with people with type 1 diabetes who aren't taking them, the benefit was generally temporary. Both groups of people were eventually given similar doses of insulin. Furthermore, these drugs have significant side-effects when used long-term, including some damage to beta cells.

  Other studies using antibodies, aimed at preserving existing beta cells, are being evaluated in newly diagnosed patients.

- ✔ **Insulin:** The theory that insulin could be used to prevent or delay the onset of type 1 diabetes dates back to 1940. Since then, a couple of small studies have provided encouraging evidence in support of this notion. As a result, a large study in the United States, the Diabetes Prevention Trial, was set up in 1994.

The first part of the study was to test whether the development of type 1 diabetes could be delayed or prevented by insulin injections. Over 300 people at high risk (50 per cent risk) of type 1 diabetes (had islet cell antibodies and low insulin levels) were randomly given either twice-daily insulin injections or were just observed. Sixty per cent of people in both groups developed diabetes, indicating that insulin injections weren't successful in preventing the onset of type 1 diabetes. The results of the second part of the study, using insulin in tablet form in people at intermediate risk (25–50 per cent) of type 1 diabetes, was also unsuccessful.

At the time of writing, an Australian study of using inhaled insulin to prevent diabetes, The Type 1 Diabetes Prevention Trial, is underway. The aim is to determine whether exposing the immune system to insulin inhaled through the nose will stop the further loss of beta cells. Because the insulin is inhaled, it doesn't cross into the bloodstream and can't cause hypoglycaemia. This study is also recruiting participants in New Zealand and Germany.

✔ **Interferon-alpha:** *Interferons* are proteins produced by the body in response to viral infections and other stimuli that are able to influence the immune system. They're currently used in clinical practice to treat chronic hepatitis B and C, chronic leukaemia and other medical problems. A study of interferon-alpha, aimed at extending the 'honeymoon phase' in humans with type 1 diabetes (refer to Chapter 3) was conducted. This study did show that low doses of this drug may prolong the honeymoon period for people with type 1 diabetes. However, the evidence is currently not robust enough to make this a standard treatment for type 1 diabetes.

✔ **Nicotinamide:** In animal studies, nicotinamide (a component of vitamin B3) protects the beta cells of mice that are diabetes-prone. Early studies in both at-risk relatives and school children with no family members with diabetes suggest that nicotinamide may delay or prevent the onset of type 1 diabetes. Doctors were surprised that a drug that may raise plasma glucose (refer to Chapter 2) could prevent diabetes. However, subsequent large European and North American studies have failed to show that nicotinamide reduces progression to diabetes in relatives of people with type 1 diabetes.

✔ **Vitamin D:** A lot of interest has recently taken place in the role of vitamin D in the development of both type 1 and type 2 diabetes. Vitamin D has anti-inflammatory effects, leading researchers to wonder whether people with low vitamin D are more susceptible to inflammatory conditions like type 1 diabetes. Studies are currently underway to determine whether vitamin D repletion will slow the progression of adult-onset autoimmune diabetes.

Avoiding Type 2 Diabetes

Type 2 diabetes is becoming a worldwide 'epidemic'. At the present time, approximately 285 million people have type 2 diabetes, and numbers are predicted to reach 438 million by 2030. At least 50 per cent of those with type 2 diabetes remain undiagnosed. In Australia, one in four adults has a disturbance in how glucose is metabolised in the body.

In Australia, levels of obesity are increasing while the amount of physical activity we do is declining. Obesity and physical inactivity are two significant lifestyle risk factors for developing type 2 diabetes. Although genetics contribute strongly to both the rise in obesity and the rise in diabetes, the escalation of these conditions appears to be due to an imbalance between energy intake and the expenditure of energy through physical exertion and activity.

The evidence is inescapable: Type 2 diabetes can certainly be delayed — and even possibly be prevented — if at-risk individuals are prepared to make changes in their lifestyles and diet, and undertake drug therapy.

Understanding the impact of diabetes on the individual and the community

While no-one will disagree that the need to prevent the onset of type 2 diabetes is a pressing one, not everyone is fully aware of the extent to which it can affect people who have it. Nor are many people outside the medical profession aware of the impact it has on Australia's health system. The impact that diabetes has on the individual and on society as a whole can be summarised as follows:

- Diabetes can cause complications and premature death, both of which can, in the main, be related to cardiovascular disease.

- Significant numbers of deaths associated with diabetes can be attributed to heart disease.

- At diagnosis, at least 50 per cent of beta cell function has already been lost, which means that this loss started many years earlier and the patient has been experiencing symptoms such as fatigue and infections. (The beta cells are those cells of the pancreas that secrete insulin; refer to Chapter 3 for further details.)

- Approximately 50 per cent of people newly diagnosed with type 2 diabetes already have one or more complications at diagnosis.

- In most developed countries, at least 10 per cent of the annual health budget is expended on diabetes and its related complications. Australia spends more than $3 billion a year on health care related to diabetes.

Modifying the lifestyle risk factors: 'The triad'

Researchers have conducted valuable studies on the prevention of type 2 diabetes, most of which confirm the benefits of increased physical activity and weight loss, as well as the benefits of using glucose-lowering drugs (namely metformin, acarbose and the thiazolidinediones). The research also suggested that people with some level of impaired glucose metabolism can certainly delay and possibly prevent the onset of diabetes, so long as they make lifestyle changes. These changes included losing 7 to 15 per cent of their body weight and increasing moderate-intensity physical activity to 150 minutes per week.

A significant finding of one study, with important implications, was that making changes in lifestyle is nearly twice as effective in prevention of developing diates as taking glucose-lowering drugs. On the other hand — but also of significance — was the study's conclusion that it's difficult to achieve these changes without intensive and costly intervention. The study's authors have now been able to assess participants 10 years after the completion of the original study. Participants in the intervention group are still enjoying a significant reduction (40 per cent) in their progression to diabetes.

Those aspects of your lifestyle that put you most at risk of contracting diabetes are ones that are totally within your ability to control. The lifestyle risk factors that you need to modify are obesity, excess kilojoule intake and reduced physical activity.

Tackling obesity

Many health surveys undertaken in developing countries report a significant increase in obesity over the past 10 to 15 years. Anyone who is overweight or obese has a significantly increased risk of developing diabetes. Chapter 11 gives detailed information on how you can calculate your body mass index, or BMI, and provides guidelines on reducing your weight.

If the escalating rates of obesity among adults are not worrying enough, even more worrying is the increase in obesity in children. Increasingly, children in developing, as well as developed countries, are contracting type 2 diabetes.

Cutting kilojoules

Over the last 50 years, our energy intake has increased somewhat while our physical activity has sharply declined (the amount of exercise that the average person takes now is almost half that their parents took). While our consumption of dietary fat has increased, we are eating less fibre, fruit and vegetables. Takeaway meals, high-energy meals that are quick to prepare, and eating on the run have replaced the eating and dining habits of an earlier generation.

Interestingly, in developed countries, type 2 diabetes is more prevalent at the lower socioeconomic levels of society than at the middle-class level (probably due to these people having a higher level of education as well as the time and/or finances to adopt a 'healthier' lifestyle), whereas in the developing countries, it is more prevalent among those at the upper socioeconomic levels (possibly related to the fact that the affluent have a higher kilojoule intake and are less active).

Getting physically active

In the United Kingdom, a study has shown that the level of adult obesity reflects the number of cars per household as well as the hours spent watching television. Studies conducted throughout the western world have also reported a marked decline in the number of people participating in organised sport or any physical activity.

Identifying at-risk individuals

High-risk groups for type 2 diabetes include people who

- ✔ Are over the age of 55
- ✔ Have cardiovascular disease
- ✔ Have a history of gestational diabetes
- ✔ Are overweight (and especially those with increased waist measurements)
- ✔ Smoke
- ✔ Have high blood pressure (hypertension)
- ✔ Have a family history of type 2 diabetes
- ✔ Are from indigenous populations
- ✔ Are from high-risk ethnic groups, such as South-East Asians, Indians and Pacific Islanders
- ✔ Have polycystic ovary disease (refer to Chapter 3)

Identifying those individuals who are most at risk is vital. Anyone who displays the signs and symptoms of diabetes should immediately consult their doctor (refer to Chapter 3).

Chapter 5

Dealing with Prediabetes

After submitting a sample of your blood for testing, your GP may tell you the sample showed a mild increase in your blood glucose levels, explaining these levels were outside the normal range but not high enough to diagnose type 2 diabetes. These mild increases have been given the name *prediabetes* and indicate an increased risk of developing type 2 diabetes, and also of developing cardiovascular disease.

In this chapter, we explain how your doctor diagnoses prediabetes, and outline which groups are most at risk. We also cover how to deal with this diagnosis and lessen the chances of future ill health, and what the diagnosis might mean for family members.

Differentiating Between Diagnoses

Prediabetes is often described as either impaired fasting glucose (IFG) or impaired glucose tolerance (IGT). These conditions are slightly different, but both diagnoses indicate that without some intervention your chance of progressing to type 2 diabetes is much higher.

Impaired fasting glucose

The diagnosis of impaired fasting glucose (IFG) can be made based on a simple blood test from your doctor. This test should be done after an overnight fast — in other words, no food or drink after midnight on the previous evening.

A fasting plasma glucose reading of 6.1 to 6.9 mmol/L means that you have impaired fasting glucose. Levels of 7 or above indicate a diagnosis of diabetes — in this case, you've already gone past the 'pre' part. The diabetes experts from the American Diabetes Association suggest that the diagnosis of IFG should be made from levels of 5.6 mmol/L upwards, but this has not yet been accepted internationally.

For this reason, if you have a blood test reading in the 'we're not sure' range — that is, between 5.6 and 6.9 mmol/L — the recommendation from the Australian Diabetes Society is that you should have an oral glucose tolerance test (OGTT) to determine whether or not you have diabetes, IFG or impaired glucose tolerance (see following section).

The OGTT is the gold standard of blood tests to determine if your pancreas can produce enough insulin.

The OGTT actually starts three days before your blood is taken. You must have a high carbohydrate diet for the three days prior to the test — so have plenty of potato, rice, bread and pasta with your meals. On the day of the test you need to have been fasting from midnight the night before. A fasting blood sample is taken, and you are then given a large, sweet, glucose-containing drink to consume. After two hours, a second blood sample is taken. By looking at both the fasting and the two-hour reading, your doctor then has the information she needs to make the correct diagnosis.

You must not go out for a walk (or anything else) during the two-hour wait between blood samples being taken for the OGTT — so bring along a good book or magazine!

After the OGTT, your doctor will diagnose you with IFG if your blood samples show the following:

- ✔ Your fasting plasma glucose reading is between 6.1 and 6.9 mmol/L
- ✔ Your follow-up two-hour level is less than 7.8 mmol/L

An important difference between IFG and impaired glucose tolerance (IGT) is that with IFG your blood glucose levels don't rise abnormally two hours after you've taken the sweet drink, while with IGT they do. IFG is more common in men.

Impaired glucose tolerance

A diagnosis of impaired glucose tolerance (IGT), which is more common in women, is made on the basis of the OGTT described in the preceding section.

After the OGTT, your doctor will diagnose you with IGT if your blood samples show the following:

✔ Your fasting plasma glucose is less than 7 mmol/L

✔ Your follow-up two-hour level is between 7.8 and 11.0 mmol/L

If your fasting level in the OGTT is above 7 or your follow-up two-hour level is above 11 mmol/L, you go straight to being diagnosed with diabetes.

Understanding these diagnoses

Being diagnosed with either IFG or IGT indicates that you have a greatly increased chance of developing type 2 diabetes; hence the term 'prediabetes'. Various studies have shown that each year 3 to 11 per cent of people with prediabetes develop diabetes. The good news is that progression to diabetes is not inevitable. When followed up some years later, approximately one-third of people with prediabetes had progressed to diabetes, one-third had remained the same and one-third had returned to normal glucose tolerance.

However, don't relax yet! Apart from the increased risk of developing diabetes, the diagnosis of prediabetes also indicates a substantially increased risk of cardiovascular disease. This relationship between abnormal blood glucose levels and cardiovascular risk is strongly associated with abdominal obesity — that is, carrying excess weight around your middle area — and has been termed 'the metabolic syndrome' (see Chapter 7).

Carrying extra weight anywhere isn't great, but it's especially not great if the weight's building up between your ribs and your hips. Men will recognise this as a 'beer gut' and women will see it as their waist disappearing (which usually coincides with a strong desire to avoid belts and embrace elasticised waistbands!).

See the sections 'Turning Back the Clock' and 'Planning For the Long Term' later in this chapter for tips on what you can do to make your risk of developing diabetes or cardiovascular disease less likely.

Knowing What Puts You at Risk

The risk factors for developing prediabetes are the same as the risk factors for developing type 2 diabetes. These include being overweight and sedentary, a smoker or someone with a family history of diabetes (refer to Chapter 4 for the full list of groups most at risk of developing type 2 diabetes).

Obviously, you can't do anything about some of these risk factors — like who your parents are — but you can modify other factors (see the following section).

Apart from a family history of diabetes, an illness of any sort, and particularly an infection, can increase the risk of prediabetes. Some medications (especially cortisone-related drugs and some medications used to treat severe mental illness) can also increase your risk of developing prediabetes (or diabetes). Ask your GP if any of your prescribed medications could increase your blood glucose levels and, if they do, get your GP to test your fasting glucose level regularly. You may not be able to stop these medications, so it is important to be screened at least once a year for diabetes so a diagnosis can be picked up as soon as possible after it occurs.

Be on the lookout for any signs of very high blood glucose levels, such as excessive thirst and increased urination, fatigue or poor healing, which could indicate your condition has progressed to diabetes. (Refer to Chapter 3 for a detailed list of the symptoms of type 2 diabetes.)

Always see your doctor if you experience any of these symptoms longer than a week or so.

Turning Back the Clock

Not everyone diagnosed with prediabetes progresses to type 2 diabetes, and some prediabetic people actually return to normal blood glucose tolerance, so turning back the clock — when it comes to prediabetes at least — is possible. In the following sections we cover the best methods for making this happen, including lifestyle changes and possible medications.

Taking on lifestyle changes

A number of studies have shown the importance of lifestyle changes in reducing your chances of progressing from prediabetes to diabetes, and even in increasing your chances of returning to normal glucose tolerance. Shown to be particularly effective were eating fewer kilojoules, losing some weight and increasing physical activity.

The two best studies involving adults with prediabetes were the American Diabetes Prevention Program and the Helsinki (Finland) Study. Amazingly, in both of these studies, people with prediabetes who made changes to their lifestyle showed exactly the same reduction — 58 per cent — in progression to diabetes. These lifestyle changes were quite modest; they included participants losing 5 to 7 per cent of their body weight and undertaking 150 to 240 minutes of moderate physical activity per week.

You don't need to lose a huge amount of weight in your bid to stop your progression to diabetes — you just need to lose some! For someone who weighs 100 kilograms, losing 5 to 7 per cent body weight equates to losing just 5 to 7 kilograms.

In both the US and the Finnish studies, participants were given detailed advice from a dietitian on lowering kilojoules (see Chapter 11 for tips on improving your diet) and increasing physical activity (see Chapter 12).

As well as losing 5 to 7 per cent body weight and increasing your daily activity to 20 to 40 minutes of moderate exercise, the following factors are also effective in turning back your diabetes 'clock':

- ✔ Reducing alcohol consumption if you currently exceed two standard drinks per day
- ✔ Reducing salt in your diet to help lower your blood pressure
- ✔ Stopping smoking

Call Quitline on 131 848 or access the federal government's Quitnow website (www.quitnow.info.au) for help on quitting smoking.

Considering medications

Researchers have found that the use of some diabetic medications may also be useful in avoiding progression from prediabetes to diabetes. These medications have been found to reduce the rate of progression to diabetes in the range of 30 to 70 per cent — not quite as good as lifestyle change!

One of the drugs used in this way has been metformin (see Chapter 10), which is at the lower end of the range in terms of effectiveness, but is the safest for long-term use.

The Australian Diabetes Society has recommended lifestyle changes alone should be the main form of treatment for prediabetes. You should only consider using medication if abnormal glucose levels persist after six months of lifestyle change.

Using metformin or other diabetic medications for prediabetes is outside the approved usage of these medications as determined by the federal government's Pharmaceutical Benefits Scheme (PBS) guidelines. This means the medications may not be available to you at the government subsidised price.

Getting the Family Involved

Prediabetes, diabetes and gestational diabetes (diabetes in pregnancy — see Chapter 18) all have a tendency to run in families. This is partly because of an increased genetic risk in related family members, but also partly because poor diet, lack of physical activity and cigarette smoking often occur in multiple family members.

In the past, a diagnosis of any type of illness was often hidden from close friends and family. However, your, and your family's, health is more important than privacy concerns. If your family has a history of diabetes, your GP needs to know about it.

As soon as you or someone in your family gets diagnosed with prediabetes (or diabetes or gestational diabetes), inform as many close family members as possible so they can also be checked. The sooner you learn of your diabetes status, the more that can be done to avoid further health problems.

Another benefit of letting your family know about your diabetes status is that the whole crowd can be then involved in taking on a healthy lifestyle, including reducing their kilojoule intake if overweight, maintaining a good level of physical activity and avoiding smoking.

Start exercising together as a family, modifying the foods you purchase at the supermarket and limiting your intake of poor-quality takeaway foods. Make water and sugar-free drinks the main thirst quenchers in your household and smoking a thing of the past. Supporting each other and making changes together can make success with lifestyle changes more likely — and more enjoyable!

 Because of the genetic links to diabetes and cardiovascular disease, if all family members get involved in making the required lifestyle changes, the benefits can be wideranging. These changes not only reduce the risk of prediabetes and diabetes but also lessen the chances of heart attack, strokes and some cancers.

Planning For the Long Term

If you are diagnosed with prediabetes, you will need to monitor your blood glucose levels, but don't worry — you don't have to start using finger-prick blood glucose testing just yet (see Chapter 9 for more on this monitoring method). You will need to do a blood test to check your fasting blood glucose level once a year, so your GP can determine whether you have progressed to type 2 diabetes and work out if further action is necessary.

 A diagnosis of prediabetes indicates an increased risk of cardiovascular problems such as heart attack and strokes. Although this risk isn't as great as in established diabetes, it's still significant — approximately twice the risk of someone without prediabetes. Therefore, it's also a good idea for you to be checked out by your GP for all the cardiovascular risk factors.

The following lists what your GP should check to monitor both your diabetes and cardiovascular wellbeing, and when:

- ✔ Blood pressure — at every visit to your GP
- ✔ Cholesterol and other blood fats — once a year
- ✔ Weight — at every visit

Perhaps not surprisingly, the lifestyle changes you can make to reduce your cardiovascular risk factors are the same as those that reduce your risk of progressing to diabetes. These include improving the quality of your diet, increasing your physical activity and quitting smoking (refer to the section 'Taking on lifestyle changes' earlier in this chapter for more information).

Part II
How Diabetes Affects Your Body

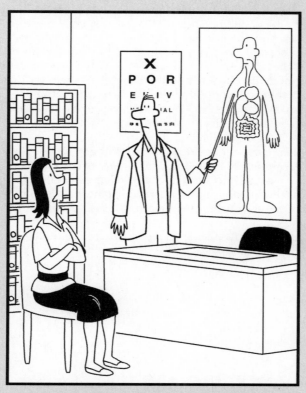

*'Maybe it'd be quicker if you listed the
bits that aren't affected by diabetes.'*

In this part ...

Diabetes, if not treated properly, can have profound effects on your body. This part explains these effects, how they occur, the kinds of symptoms they produce, and what you and your doctor need to do to treat them. You may be surprised at how many parts of your body can be affected by diabetes. Remember that many things described in this part are preventable — and even if you haven't been able to prevent diabetes, it is very treatable.

Medical research has resulted in great advances in the treatment of diabetes. While many of the effects of the disease may be reduced or even eliminated in the not-too-distant future, it's important that you know about the effects and respond to them appropriately.

Chapter 6

Managing the Lumps and Bumps of Day-to-Day Diabetes

· ·

In This Chapter

▶ Understanding the complications involved with short-term illness

▶ Managing your health while battling colds and other sicknesses

▶ Dealing with low blood glucose

▶ Handling very high blood glucose

▶ Coping with the highest blood glucose

· ·

C hapters 2 and 3 tell you how doctors make a diagnosis of diabetes and how they determine which type of diabetes you have. Those chapters cover some of the signs and symptoms of diabetes, which you could consider to be the shortest of the short-term problems of the disease because they're generally mild and begin to subside when you start treatment. This chapter covers the more serious forms of short-term issues of diabetes management, which occur when your blood glucose is out of control — reaching uncomfortably high or low levels. We refer to these events as the 'lumps and bumps of diabetes'.

With the exception of mild *hypoglycaemia* (low blood glucose) or mild *ketoacidosis* (high blood glucose) you should treat all the complications described in this chapter as medical emergencies. Keep in touch with your doctor or diabetes educator when the symptoms are mild, and go to hospital promptly if your blood glucose is uncontrollably high or you're unable to hold down food. You may need a few hours in the emergency department or a day or two in hospital to reverse your problems.

Solving Short-Term Problems

Although the problems covered in this chapter are called *short term*, you may experience them at any time during the course of your diabetes. *Short term* simply means that these conditions arise rapidly in your body, as opposed to the long-term complications that take years to develop. (See Chapter 7 for the details of long-term complications.) Short-term problems develop in days or even hours and, fortunately, they respond to treatment just as rapidly.

The short-term problems of diabetes like low blood glucose levels (hypoglycaemia) may affect your ability to function normally. You may find that the authority that governs road safety and driver licensing in your state (such as the Road Transport Authority in New South Wales or VicRoads in Victoria) and the Civil Aviation Safety Authority (CASA) are more careful about giving you, and all people with diabetes, a driver's licence or a pilot's licence. Potential employers may question your ability to perform certain jobs. But most companies and government departments are very enlightened about diabetes and do everything possible to accommodate you in these situations. (Chapter 19 shows you how to overcome challenges you may face with employment and insurance. Contact the Australian Diabetes Council (in NSW) or Diabetes Australia in other states or territories if you feel that you have been discriminated against because of your diabetes.)

You don't have to feel limited in what you can do. You can have control over your diabetes, and all the short-term problems are manageable. If you closely monitor and control your blood glucose, you can quickly determine any drop to lower than normal levels or elevations to higher than normal levels, and you can treat these problems before they affect your mental and physical functioning. (See Chapter 9 for all details on glucose monitoring and other testing.)

Coping With Colds and Other Nasties

Everyone comes down with a mild illness or virus once in a while. For most people, even those with diabetes, these illnesses cause them some inconvenience and maybe a few days away from work. However for some people with diabetes, even a mild illness can cause problems with their blood glucose levels.

When you are unwell with a virus such as the common cold, your immune system is fighting madly to destroy the virus and make you well again. Stress hormones are also increased at this time and these can make your body more resistant to insulin, which makes your blood glucose levels rise. They may rise a little or quite a lot — each illness is slightly different.

In the following sections, we cover ways you can manage your health while sick with minor illnesses, and highlight what you need to be most aware of.

Your diabetes care team may refer to the occasions of illness as 'sick days' and can discuss strategies for sick-day management with you.

Being prepared for sick days

When you come down with a virus like the common cold or influenza, you hardly feel at the top of your game, so it pays to know how to cope with illness *before* you get sick.

If you have a short-term illness you should

- **Get plenty of rest**

- **Drink plenty of fluids** — sugar free if your blood glucose levels are normal or high; sweet if your blood glucose levels are low

- **Eat a little and often** — avoid spicy and fatty foods, especially if you have an upset stomach

- **Keep taking your insulin or tablets** — even if you're hardly eating, continue to take your prescribed medications because your body still needs them all

- **Contact your doctor if the illness persists** — call your GP if you're still feeling sick after a few days or if you seem to be getting worse rather than better

Put together a 'sick day' kit that contains a range of items for when you're unwell, and keep it stocked up and easily accessible.

Here's a list of items to keep in your sick day kit:

- Blood glucose and ketone test strips (check they're not past their expiry dates)

- Cans of lemonade (or equivalent)

- Contact details of your local doctor, endocrinologist, local diabetes centre, and/or after-hours medical service

- Pain relief

- Sachets of oral rehydration solution

- Sick Day information booklet (published by the Australian Diabetes Educators Association and available from your diabetes team)

- Small packet of plain biscuits, such as crackers or sweet biscuits

- Thermometer

Monitoring glucose

When battling illness, many people with diabetes monitor their blood glucose levels less frequently because they 'know it will be high anyway' or 'just feel too sick to test'. Unfortunately, failing to monitor your glucose levels when unwell can make things worse.

If you have type 2 diabetes, continue to test at your usual frequency (see Chapter 9 for more on blood glucose and other testing). If you notice that the levels are getting higher, start to test more often to see if there is a new pattern to your blood glucose levels.

If you have type 1 diabetes, increase your frequency of testing because, when you're sick, things can go haywire quite quickly. Missing food may cause you to have hypoglycaemia, or the illness itself may make your glucose levels rise significantly. The more often you test, the quicker you will be able to sort out any problems.

When unwell, people with type 1 diabetes more commonly record high blood glucose levels (hyperglycaemia), rather than low blood glucose levels (hypoglycaemia), even if not eating.

If you're testing your blood glucose levels and regularly getting levels greater than 14 mmol/L, or you have a significant increase in your thirst or urination, contact your doctor or diabetes service for advice.

Observing ketones

If you have type 1 diabetes and are battling a minor illness, as well as monitoring your blood glucose levels (see preceding section) you should also be aware of your ketone levels. (If you have type 2 diabetes, just monitoring your blood glucose levels is fine, so feel free to skip this section!)

Having type 1 diabetes means your body is totally reliant on the insulin you inject. While higher blood glucose levels are the first indication your body needs more insulin, another sign is when your body switches to burning fat instead of glucose for energy. As the body burns up fat, it produces a rather nasty by-product called *ketones*. A raised level of ketones in your blood can make you feel worse, so always check your ketone levels when you're unwell. (See Chapter 9 for more on testing for ketones).

Knowing what to eat and drink

As someone with diabetes, you've probably been told how important it is to eat regular meals. However, when you're sick, you might not be interested in food at all — or, worse, you might have a nasty diarrhoea and vomiting bug, and can't keep much down. Don't worry — illness isn't your usual state, so the requirement to eat regular meals doesn't necessarily apply. What becomes most important is that you drink plenty of fluids throughout the day.

Our bodies absorb fluids containing small amounts of sugar and salt better than plain water alone, so drink a mixture of slightly sweet fluids, such as weak cordial or diluted fruit juice, and slightly salty fluids, such as clear broth or consommé or Vegemite mixed with hot water. Alternatively, you can use sachets of oral re-hydration solution (available from the chemist) to make drinks or iceblocks.

Drink small amounts often. Drinking 250 millilitres should take you about one hour.

If you feel ready for something more solid, try dry crackers or toast. Avoid margarine or butter (these fats can make nausea worse), and go for foods that have little or no smell. Progress back to your usual diet as your body tells you.

Contacting important people

Managing your blood glucose levels when you're feeling unwell can be difficult — particularly if it's the first time you've been sick since being diagnosed with diabetes. And while having a poor intake of food will cause little damage to your body over only a few days, the lack of food becomes more troublesome if a short-term illness turns into something more serious and long term.

If your blood glucose levels are rising, you're not getting better and/or your ketones are high, call your GP or diabetes care team. Some advice and reassurance from them may be all that you need, and they can also assist you in managing the situation at home — or they may recommend a trip to the hospital if they believe the situation is more serious. If it's out-of-hours, go to the emergency department of your local hospital or call the after-hours line for your local diabetes centre.

Understanding Hypoglycaemia

The condition of low blood glucose is known as *hypoglycaemia*. If you have diabetes, you can get hypoglycaemia only as a consequence of your diabetes treatment.

As a person with diabetes, you're in constant combat with *high* blood glucose, which is responsible for most of the long-term and short-term complications of the disease. Your doctor prescribes drugs and other treatments in an effort to finetune your blood glucose as it would be in someone else's body. (Part III explains many techniques that help you to control your blood glucose levels.) But, unfortunately, these drugs and treatments aren't always perfect. If you take too much of a drug, exercise too much or eat too little, or you become suddenly unwell, your blood glucose can drop to the low levels at which symptoms develop — and this can occur in both type 1 and type 2 diabetes. The following sections explain more about hypoglycaemia's symptoms, causes and treatment.

Getting acquainted with the signs and symptoms

Your body doesn't function well when you have too little glucose in your blood. Your brain needs glucose to run the rest of your body, as well as for intellectual purposes. Your muscles need the energy that glucose provides in much the same way that your car needs petrol. So, when your body detects that it has low blood glucose, it sends out a group of hormones that rapidly raise your glucose. But those hormones have to fight the strength of the diabetes medication that has been pushing down your glucose levels.

At what level of blood glucose do you develop hypoglycaemia? Unfortunately, the level varies for different individuals, particularly depending on the length of time that the person has had diabetes. But most experts agree that a blood glucose of 4.0 mmol/L or less is associated with signs and symptoms of hypoglycaemia in most people.

If you have too many episodes of hypoglycaemia (more likely if you have type 1 diabetes), you can lose the early symptoms of hypoglycaemia. If these early warning signs no longer appear, you can progress quickly to altered consciousness or even unconsciousness.

Doctors traditionally put the symptoms of hypoglycaemia into two major categories:

✔ **Symptoms that are due to your brain not receiving enough fuel so that your intellectual function suffers.** This first category of symptoms is called *neuroglycopaenic* symptoms, which is medical talk for 'not enough (*paenic*) glucose (*glyco*) in the brain (*neuro*)'. (If your brain could speak, it would just say, 'Whew, I'm ready for a meal!')

✔ **Symptoms due to the side effects of the hormones (especially adrenaline) that your body sends out to counter the glucose-lowering effect of insulin.** The second category of symptoms is called *adrenergic* symptoms, because adrenaline, a stress hormone, comes from your adrenal gland.

Adrenergic symptoms occur most often when your blood glucose falls rapidly. These symptoms are often the first sign of hypoglycaemia, and serve as a warning that you need to check your glucose level and treat yourself if it is low.

The following adrenergic symptoms may warn you that you're hypoglycaemic:

✔ Anxiety

✔ Palpitations, or the feeling that your heart is beating too fast

✔ Rapid heartbeat

✔ Sensation of hunger

✔ Sweating

✔ Whiteness, or pallor, of your skin

Neuroglycopaenic symptoms occur most often when your hypoglycaemia takes longer to develop. The symptoms become more severe as your blood glucose drops lower and you will require urgent medical attention. The following neuroglycopaenic symptoms are often signs that you're becoming (or already are) hypoglycaemic:

✔ Coma, or an inability to be awakened

✔ Confusion

✔ Convulsions

✔ Fatigue

✔ Headache

✔ Loss of concentration

✔ Visual disorders, such as double vision

People lose their ability to think clearly when they become hypoglycaemic. They make simple mistakes, and other people often assume that they are drunk.

One of our patients was driving on a freeway when a police officer noticed that she was weaving back and forth in her lane and pulled her over. He concluded that she was drunk and took her to the police station. Fortunately, someone noticed that she was wearing a medical alert bracelet engraved with her diabetes details. After promptly receiving the nutrition that she needed, she rapidly recovered. No charges were laid, but clearly this is a situation that you want to avoid. Always test your blood glucose level to make sure that it's satisfactory before driving your car.

If you take insulin or a *sulphonylurea drug,* which squeezes more insulin out of your reluctant pancreas, for your own safety you need to wear or carry with you some form of identification, in case you unexpectedly develop hypoglycaemia. You should also carry with you information regarding your diagnosis, a list of your current medications and the contact details for your doctor or a family member, in case you are unable to communicate. (See Chapter 10 for a full explanation of the insulin and sulphonylurea medications.)

Knowing the causes

Hypoglycaemia results from elevated amounts of insulin driving down your blood glucose to low levels, but an extra high dose of insulin or sulphonylurea isn't always the culprit that elevates your insulin level. The amount of food you take in, the amount of fuel (glucose) that you burn for energy, the amount of insulin circulating in your body and your body's ability to raise glucose by releasing it from the liver or making it from other body substances all affect your blood glucose level.

Insulin and sulphonylurea drugs

When you have insulin injections, you have to time your food intake to raise your blood glucose as the insulin is taking effect. Chapter 10 explains the different kinds of insulin and the proper methods for administering them. But remember that the different types of insulin are most potent at differing amounts of time (minutes or hours) after you inject them. If you miss a meal or take your insulin too early or too late, your glucose and insulin levels won't be in sync and you'll develop hypoglycaemia. If you go on a diet and don't adjust your medication, the same thing happens.

When taking insulin, mistakes can happen. Sometimes hypoglycaemia results from taking the wrong dose or the wrong type of insulin, so even if you've been taking insulin for many years, still double-check what you are taking every time you take it.

If you take sulphonylurea drugs, you need to follow similar precautions. You and your doctor must adjust your dosage when your kilojoule intake falls. Other drugs, such as metformin, don't cause hypoglycaemia by themselves, but when combined with sulphonylureas they may lower your glucose enough to reach hypoglycaemic levels. (Chapter 10 talks more about these other drugs.)

Diet

Your diet plays a major role in helping you to avoid hypoglycaemia if you take medication. You will usually need to eat breakfast, lunch and dinner at regular times each day.

When you need to eat meals, and how much you should eat at each meal, differs depending on the type of insulin you take. Always discuss your need (or lack thereof) for meals and snacks with your diabetes dietitian when starting insulin or changing the type or dose you take.

Most people with type 2 diabetes don't need to eat snacks to prevent hypoglycaemia. If you're regularly experiencing hypoglycaemia, discuss this situation with your GP, endocrinologist or diabetes care team — it may be your medication that needs adjustment, rather than your diet.

Chapter 11 gives much greater detail about how you can best manage your individual dietary needs.

Exercise

Exercise burns more of your body's fuel, which is glucose, so it generally lowers your blood glucose. Some people with diabetes use exercise in place of extra insulin to get their high blood glucose down to a normal level. However, if you don't adjust your insulin dose or food intake to match your exercise, exercise can result in hypoglycaemia.

People who exercise regularly require much less medication and generally can manage their diabetes more easily than non-exercisers can. Talk to your diabetes care team about how best to fit exercise into your life. (See Chapter 12 for more on the benefits of exercise.)

Non-diabetes medications

Several drugs that you may take unrelated to your diabetes can lower your blood glucose. One important and widely used drug, which you may not even think of as a drug, is alcohol (in the form of wine, beer and spirits). Alcohol can block your liver's ability to release glucose. It also blocks hormones that raise blood glucose and increases the glucose-lowering effect of insulin. If you drink alcohol on an empty stomach, in the evening or before going to bed, you may experience severe hypoglycaemia overnight or the next morning. While this is more common in those people with type 1 diabetes, those with type 2 may also notice this effect.

Watch out for these drugs that can lower your blood glucose:

- **Alcohol:** If you take insulin or sulphonylurea drugs, don't drink alcohol without eating some food at the same time. Food counteracts some of the glucose-lowering effects of alcohol.

- **Aspirin:** On rare occasions aspirin (and all the drugs related to aspirin, called *salicylates*) can lead you to hypoglycaemia if used in high doses (greater than 300 milligrams per day). In adults who have diabetes, aspirin can increase the effects of other drugs that you're taking to lower your blood glucose. In children with diabetes, aspirin has an especially profound effect on lowering blood glucose to hypoglycaemia levels.

Treating the problem

The vast majority of hypoglycaemia cases are mild. If you (or a friend or relative) notice that you have the early symptoms of hypoglycaemia, you can treat the problem with a small quantity of glucose in the form of

- Pre-packaged sachet of glucose gel
- Three small sugar cubes or sachets
- Three glucose tablets (available from chemists)
- Six to eight jelly beans
- 150 millilitres (or about half a cup) of a sugary soft drink or fruit juice

Sometimes you need a second treatment. Approximately ten minutes after you try one of these solutions, measure your blood glucose to find out whether your level has risen sufficiently. If it is still low, again take one of the forms of glucose in the preceding list.

This fast-acting glucose only lasts a short time, and it's important that within the next hour you eat another small serve of a carbohydrate source such as a piece of fruit, a slice of bread or two plain sweet biscuits, in addition to the initial glucose treatment, in order to prevent further lowering of blood glucose levels. Continue to monitor your glucose levels and watch for further signs of hypoglycaemia, as some insulins can have a long duration of effect.

Because your mental state may be mildly confused when you have hypoglycaemia, you need to make sure that your friends or relatives know in advance what hypoglycaemia is and what to do about it. Inform people about your diabetes and about how to recognise hypoglycaemia. Don't keep your diabetes a secret. The people close to you will be glad to know how to help you.

If you can't sit up and swallow properly when you have hypoglycaemia, people shouldn't try to feed you, as this may cause more harm. Instead, use one of the following options:

- **A subcutaneous or intramuscular injection of glucagon (1 mg, equivalent to 1 international unit) into your outer thigh.** Glucagon is one of the major hormones that raise glucose levels. The injection of glucagon raises your blood glucose so that you regain consciousness within 20 minutes and then corrects your hypoglycaemic condition for about an hour, so you must eat or drink some carbohydrate-containing food when you can swallow properly. You need to get a prescription from your doctor for the glucagon kit, which includes instructions on its administration. Make sure that a friend or relative reads these instructions. Also make sure that the kit doesn't become outdated if you haven't used it for a long time.

- **An emergency 000 call.** If your hypoglycaemia recurs shortly after you receive glucagon or doesn't respond to the glucagon, the person helping you needs to make an emergency 000 call. The ambulance officers check your blood glucose and give you an intravenous (IV) dose of high-concentration glucose. Most likely, you will continue the IV in the emergency department until you show stable and normal blood glucose levels.

After a case of hypoglycaemia — and after the sweat has dried and the shakes have gone — it's a good idea to sit down and think about why this condition might have occurred. Could it have been related to food, alcohol, exercise or incorrect insulin dose? Or are you just not sure? Contact your GP or diabetes care team to discuss possible causes of your hypoglycaemia and how you can prevent it happening again.

Combating Diabetic Ketoacidosis

Chapter 3 talks about the tendency of people with type 1 diabetes to develop a severe complication called *ketoacidosis*, or very high blood glucose with large amounts of acid in the blood.

 The prefix *keto* refers to *ketones* — substances that your body makes as fat breaks down during ketoacidosis. *Acid* is part of the name because your blood becomes acidic from the presence of ketones. Ketoacidosis can be the symptom that tells doctors that you have type 1 diabetes, but more frequently it occurs after you already know that you have the disease.

Ketoacidosis occurs mostly in people with type 1 diabetes because they have no insulin in their bodies except what they inject as medication. Those with type 2 diabetes (or with other forms of the disease) rarely develop ketoacidosis (although it is possible), because they have some insulin in their bodies, even though the insulin usually isn't fully active due to insulin resistance. People with type 2 diabetes get something similar to ketoacidosis usually when they have severe infections or traumas that put their bodies under great physical stress (see the section 'Managing Hyperglycaemic Hyperosmolar State' later in this chapter).

The following sections explain symptoms, causes and treatments of ketoacidosis.

Recognising the symptoms

The symptoms of ketoacidosis regularly alert doctors to a new diagnosis of type 1 diabetes in both children and adults. However, ketoacidosis can also occur at other times during your life with diabetes, so keep an eye out for the following symptoms:

- **Nausea and vomiting:** You experience these symptoms because of the build-up of acids and the loss of important body substances.

- **Rapid deep breathing:** (This is also known as *Kussmaul breathing*, after the man who first described it.) You experience rapid deep breathing when your blood is so acidic that your body attempts to blow off some of the acid through the lungs. Your breath has a fruity smell due to acetone.

- **Extreme tiredness and drowsiness:** You're tired because your brain is bathed in very thick blood, like syrup, and is missing the essential substances you've lost in the urine.

- **Weakness:** You become weak because your muscle tissue is unable to get its fuel, namely glucose.

In this age of self-monitoring for blood glucose levels, ketoacidosis is becoming rarer, but it does still occur. (See Chapter 9 for information on self-monitoring.) If you use a source of insulin that can be interrupted, you could unexpectedly develop ketoacidosis. For example, if you rely on an insulin pump, which pushes insulin under your skin automatically (as described in Chapter 10), the pump could stop; then your insulin delivery would cease, your glucose level would rise and ketoacidosis would develop if you didn't notice the interruption soon enough. Interruption of insulin can also occur due to missed doses, or insulin being out of date or not effective, which can happen especially during hot weather.

Doctors make a diagnosis of ketoacidosis when they see the following abnormalities, some of which you will also be able to identify:

- ✔ High blood glucose, usually more than 16.6 mmol/L
- ✔ Acid condition of your blood (which may make you feel short of breath)
- ✔ Excessive levels of ketones in your blood and/or urine
- ✔ Dry skin and tongue, indicating dehydration
- ✔ Deficiency of potassium in your body
- ✔ An acetone smell on your breath

See the section 'Dealing with ketoacidosis' for more on treatment of this condition.

Identifying the causes

The most common causes of ketoacidosis are interruption of your insulin treatment or an infection. Your body can't go for many hours without insulin before it begins to burn fat for energy and begins to make extra glucose that it can't use. The process of burning fat creates ketones in your blood, which are responsible for your ketoacidosis.

If you go on a strict diet to lose weight, your body burns some of its fat stores and produces ketones, similar to how it burns fat when you lack insulin. But in this case, your glucose remains low and (unless you have type 1 diabetes) you have sufficient insulin to prevent excessive production of new glucose or release of large amounts of glucose from your liver. So a strict diet doesn't generally lead to ketoacidosis.

Dealing with ketoacidosis

Ketoacidosis is a serious condition that requires prompt treatment. The basis of ketoacidosis treatment is to restore the proper amount of water to your body, reduce the acid condition of your blood by getting rid of the ketones, restore substances such as potassium that you've lost and return your blood glucose to its normal levels. All these improvements should happen simultaneously after you begin treatment.

You *can* manage mild episodes of ketoacidosis at home, without needing to go into hospital. (A mild episode of ketoacidosis does *not* involve vomiting, abdominal pain or shortness of breath. Your blood ketone levels are less than 1.5 mmol/L, or your urine ketones show moderate, negative or trace results when tested. You're also not becoming progressively more ill.) Discuss a ketoacidosis treatment plan with your doctor or diabetes care team and then have it written down to refer to when necessary.

Your treatment plan will tell you when you need to

- ✔ Take more insulin
- ✔ Monitor your blood glucose and ketone levels more frequently (see Chapter 9 for more on testing these levels)
- ✔ Drink plenty of fluids
- ✔ Rest and take it easy
- ✔ Contact your diabetes care team (your treatment plan should also include the best way to contact your team)

The amount of extra insulin people require varies so this should be at the top of your list to discuss with your doctor or diabetes care team. Keep the details of your insulin requirements with your ketoacidosis treatment plan.

If your home treatment plan isn't successful and a mild case of ketoacidosis has become more serious, you may require hospital admission. Signs your condition has become more serious include when you have vomited more than a couple of times and can't seem to keep anything down or your treatment strategies are not working and your blood glucose or ketone levels are rising. (Refer to the earlier section 'Recognising the symptoms' for the full list of the warning signs for ketoacidosis.)

After you're admitted to hospital, your doctor sets up a flow chart to keep track of your levels of glucose, acid, potassium and ketones, along with other parameters. Although you've lost a lot of potassium, for example, the initial blood reading of potassium on your flow chart may look normal.

As your treatment progresses, more potassium goes into your cells to replenish losses there, so your blood potassium may fall. If that happens, the doctor administers more potassium to fix the problem.

Obviously, because your lack of insulin got you into this ketoacidosis situation, your doctor gives you insulin intravenously to restore your insulin levels and reverse the abnormalities in your body. At some point, your blood glucose may fall towards hypoglycaemia. If it does, your doctor gives you another IV made up of glucose and a solution of salt, potassium and water.

After you receive insulin, your body stops breaking down fat for energy because your cells can use glucose for energy as they're supposed to. Soon, your body rids itself of the ketones in your bloodstream that caused your complication and your body returns to a more normal condition.

Your doctor gives you large volumes of a saltwater solution intravenously to replace the large volume of fluids that you lose during ketoacidosis. Replenishing your body's fluids relieves the nausea and vomiting that you've endured, and you're now able to keep down liquid and solid foods again. You should notice your normal mental functioning returning, which means that you'll soon be ready to resume self-administering your insulin and controlling your own diet. By this time, the doctor has probably found and corrected a malfunctioning insulin pump or an infection that was a factor in causing your ketoacidosis.

Children with type 1 diabetes develop ketoacidosis more rapidly than adults. If your child with diabetes is unwell, monitor your child regularly and carefully, and immediately contact your diabetes care team, local hospital or ambulance service if you're concerned or if your child's condition deteriorates.

Ketoacidosis may not sound like a walk in the park, but you may think that your doctor can control it with little or no risk to you. For the most part, that's true, but be aware that ketoacidosis can be fatal for a small percentage of people with diabetes who get it — mostly elderly people with diabetes and those with other illnesses that complicate treatment. Recognising the symptoms early and seeking treatment quickly greatly enhance your chances of an uneventful recovery from ketoacidosis.

If you're unfortunate enough to experience ketoacidosis, you quickly find out how unpleasant and potentially dangerous it can be. If it does happen to you, reflect on what may have gone wrong in your self-management regime to have caused the problem. Talk to your doctor or diabetes care team about modifying your ketoacidosis treatment plan just in case there is a 'next time'.

Managing Hyperglycaemic Hyperosmolar State

In people with type 2 diabetes, high blood glucose levels can lead you to a condition known as *hyperglycaemic hyperosmolar state* (HHS). This condition is a medical emergency that needs to be treated in a hospital.

In HHS, your blood glucose level is raised considerably higher than with ketoacidosis but ketoacidosis isn't present because enough insulin is still present to inhibit the breakdown of fat.

The term *hyperglycaemic hyperosmolar state* refers to the excessive levels of glucose in the blood. *Hyper* means 'larger than normal', and *osmolar* has to do with concentrations of substances in the blood. So hyperosmolar, in this situation, means that the blood is simply too concentrated with glucose. Other hyperosmolar syndromes occur when other substances are at fault.

The following sections explain the symptoms, causes and treatments for HHS.

Seeing the symptoms

HHS has some of the same symptoms as ketoacidosis. An important difference is that with HHS, you don't experience the rapid Kussmaul breathing, because your blood isn't overly acidic as a part of this complication. Also, the symptoms of HHS develop over many days or weeks, and can be mild, unlike ketoacidosis's quick and acute development in your body.

If you measure your blood glucose on a daily basis, you should never develop HHS because you'll notice that your blood glucose is getting high before it reaches a critical level.

The most important signs and symptoms of HHS are as follows:

- ✔ Blood glucose of 33.3 mmol/L, or even higher if you wait too long to seek medical help
- ✔ Decreased mental awareness or coma
- ✔ Frequent urination
- ✔ Leg cramps

- Sunken eyeballs and rapid pulse, due to dehydration
- Thirst
- Weakness

You may also develop more threatening symptoms with this complication. Your blood pressure may be low and your nervous system may be affected with paralysis of the arms and legs, but both conditions respond to treatment. You may have high counts of potassium, sodium and other blood constituents (such as white blood cells and red blood cells). With treatment these counts usually fall rapidly and your doctor will replace these elements in your blood as water is restored to your body. Treatment needs to start quickly, however, so seek medical assistance immediately if you experience more than one of the symptoms in the preceding list.

Finding the causes

HHS is more likely to occur in people with diabetes who live alone or in those whose diabetes hasn't been carefully monitored. These people may have mild type 2 diabetes that perhaps has been previously undiagnosed and/or untreated.

Age is also a contributing cause of HHS because your kidneys gradually become less efficient as you age. When your kidneys are in their prime, your blood glucose level needs to reach only 10 mmol/L before your kidneys begin to remove some excess glucose through your urine. But as your kidneys grow older and slower, they require a gradually higher blood glucose level before they start to send excess glucose to your urine. If you're at an age (usually 70 or older for people in average health) when your kidneys are really labouring to remove the excess glucose from your body and you happen to lose a large amount of fluids from sickness or neglect, your blood volume decreases, which makes it even harder for your kidneys to remove glucose. At this point, your blood glucose level begins to skyrocket. If you don't replace some of the lost fluids soon, your glucose rises even higher.

If you allow your blood glucose to rise and you don't get the fluids you need, your blood pressure starts to fall and you get weaker and weaker. As the concentration of glucose in your blood continues to rise, you become increasingly confused. Your mental state diminishes as the glucose concentration rises until you eventually fall into a coma.

Other factors — such as infection, failure to take your insulin, and taking certain medications — can raise your blood glucose to HHS levels; however, not replacing lost body fluids is the most frequent cause.

Remedying hyperglycaemic hyperosmolar state

HSS requires immediate and skilled treatment from a doctor. By no means should you try to treat HHS yourself. You need the proper treatment from an experienced doctor — and you need it fast. The death rate for HHS is high because many of the people who develop it are elderly and often have other serious illnesses that complicate treatment.

When you arrive at your doctor's surgery or at the emergency department with HSS, your doctor must accomplish the following tasks fairly rapidly:

- ✔ Restore large volumes of water to your body
- ✔ Lower your blood glucose level
- ✔ Restore other substances that your body has lost, such as potassium, sodium, chloride, and so on

Your doctor creates a chart to monitor your levels of glucose, blood concentration (osmolarity), potassium, sodium and other tests, which are measured hourly in some cases. You may think that you need to receive large amounts of insulin to lower your high glucose level, but the large doses of fluids that your doctor gives you do so much to lower your glucose that you need only smaller doses of insulin. As your body fluids return to normal, your kidneys begin to receive much more of the blood that they need in order to rid your body of the excess glucose.

If you're unfortunate enough to experience HHS, after you have recovered, consider which factors may have caused the problem and how you can avoid it happening again. For example, did you stop testing your blood glucose levels, stop taking your tablets or put off seeing your doctor when feeling unwell? Discuss possible causes with your doctor and diabetes care team.

Chapter 7

Preventing Long-Term Complications

. . . .

In This Chapter

▶ Encountering long-term complications

▶ Dealing with kidney disease

▶ Handling problems with your eyes

▶ Battling damage to your nerves

▶ Understanding the effects of diabetes on your heart

▶ Keeping your cholesterol under control

▶ Rectifying problems with sexual function

▶ Identifying skin complaints

. . . .

Complications can occur if your blood glucose rises and remains high over many years. The point that we stress throughout this book is that you have a choice: If you work with your doctor and diabetes care team, we can help you can keep your blood glucose near normal, and you may never have to deal with any long-term complications.

The most important study of prevention ever undertaken for type 1 diabetes is called the Diabetes Control and Complications Trial (DCCT), published in 1993. The DCCT showed that keeping very tight control over your blood glucose is possible but difficult. The difficult part in keeping your blood glucose close to normal is that you increase your risk of having low blood glucose, or hypoglycaemia (refer to Chapter 6). Further follow-up with this group in recent years has only strengthened the evidence for the ongoing benefits of good control of blood glucose levels.

Two types of complications are associated with long-term poor blood glucose control: *Microvascular* disease, which affects the eyes, kidneys and nerves, and *macrovascular* disease, which affects the heart and other major blood vessels, such as those to the legs and the brain.

The DCCT showed that if you already suffered from long-term complications, improving your blood glucose control very significantly slowed the progression of the complications. Since the DCCT, doctors generally treat diabetes by keeping the patient's blood glucose as close to normal as possible and practical.

How Long-Term Complications Develop

Apart from heart disease, doctors believe that years of high blood glucose levels initiate most of the long-term complications of diabetes — such as kidney disease, eye disease and nerve disease. (In the case of heart disease, high blood glucose levels may make the disease worse or more complicated but not actually cause it.) Most long-term complications require five or more years to develop, which seems like a long time until you consider that many people with type 2 diabetes have had it for five or more years before a doctor diagnoses it.

Often the long-term complication itself (rather than a high blood glucose level) is the clue that leads a doctor to diagnose type 2 diabetes in a patient. Doctors need to look for long-term complications immediately after diagnosing type 2 diabetes, because the patient may have been suffering from diabetes and its long-term complications for some time already. Because of this possibility, your doctor must immediately take steps to control your glucose levels.

How high glucose leads to complications

Doctors aren't certain about the causes of most long-term complications of diabetes, but it's an active area of research. Other pathways by which high glucose levels can add to tissue damage are being evaluated.

We mention current theories about the causes of the complications as we explain each of the complication in the sections of this chapter.

As well as the specific causes, all long-term complications share several common characteristics, as follows:

✔ **Advanced glycated (glycosylated) end products (AGEs) can damage tissues.** AGEs can damage the eyes, the kidneys, the nervous system and other organs in your body. You always have glucose in your blood, and some of that glucose attaches to other substances in your bloodstream to form *glycated* (glucose-attached) products. In this way, haemoglobin, which carries oxygen through your blood to cells and tissues throughout your body, attaches to glucose to form *haemoglobin A1c. Albumin*, a protein in blood, forms glycated albumin. Glucose can attach to red blood cells and white blood cells as well as to other cells and molecules in the bloodstream. When these normal body substances attach to glucose, they no longer work normally.

✔ **When glucose attaches to other substances and cells, it alters their functions, usually in a negative fashion.** For example, haemoglobin A1c holds on to oxygen more strongly than haemoglobin, so the cells that need oxygen don't get it as easily. Red blood cells that are glycated don't last as long in your blood circulation. Glycated white blood cells can't fight infection as well as unglycated white cells can. Your body handles a certain level of glycated substances, but when your blood glucose is elevated for prolonged periods of time, the level of glycated cells and substances becomes excessive, and the complications we describe in this chapter result.

✔ **The Polyol Pathway can damage the body in diabetes.** The *Polyol Pathway* refers to one direction, or pathway, that glucose can take as it's *metabolised* (broken down). For example, the common pathway is to form carbon dioxide and water as energy is produced. When you have a lot of glucose in your blood, an abnormal amount is metabolised to become a product called *sorbitol*. Sorbitol is a member of a class of substances called *polyols*. Sorbitol accumulates in many tissues where it can damage them in various ways:

- **Damage from swelling:** Body water enters the cells to make the concentration of substances equal outside and inside, because sorbitol doesn't pass out of the cell. This causes damage and destruction of cells.

- **Damage from chemical reactions:** During the production of sorbitol, other compounds are produced that chemically damage the cells and tissues.

Controlling Kidney Disease

Your kidneys rid your body of many harmful chemicals and other compounds produced during the process of normal metabolism. Your kidneys act like a filter through which your blood pours, trapping the waste and sending it out in your urine, while the normal contents of the blood go back into your bloodstream. Kidneys also regulate the salt and water content of your body. When kidney disease (also known as *nephropathy*) causes your kidneys to fail, you must either use artificial means, called *dialysis*, to cleanse your blood and control the salt and water, or you may receive a new working donor kidney, called a *transplant*.

In Australia, around a quarter of the patients who require long-term dialysis require it because of diabetes. Fortunately, this number is on the decline because of the increasing awareness among people that they need to control their blood glucose. Although the incidence of kidney disease is higher among people with type 1 diabetes than type 2, the absolute number of patients with kidney disease is about the same for the two groups, because type 2 diabetes is about ten times as common as type 1.

Diabetes and your kidneys

Your kidneys contain a structure called the *glomerulus*, which is responsible for cleansing your blood (see Figure 7-1). Each kidney has hundreds of thousands of glomeruli. Your blood passes through the tiny glomerular capillaries, which are in intimate contact with tubules through which your filtered blood travels. As the filtered blood passes through the tubules, most of the water and the normal contents of the blood are reabsorbed and sent back into your body, while a small amount of water and waste passes from the kidney into the ureter and then into the bladder and out through the urethra.

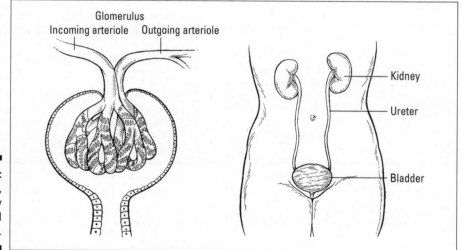

Figure 7-1:
The kidney, internally and externally.

The more rapid transit of blood through the kidneys when your blood glucose levels are high is known as an increased *glomerular filtration rate* (GFR). Early in the development of your diabetes, the membrane surrounding your glomeruli, called the *glomerular basement membrane*, thickens, as do other adjacent structures. These expanding membranes and structures begin to take up the space occupied by the capillaries inside the glomeruli so that the capillaries are unable to filter as much blood.

Fortunately, you have many more glomeruli than you really need. In fact, you can lose a whole kidney and still have plenty of reserve to clean your blood. However, if your kidney disease goes undetected for about 15 years, damage may become so severe that your blood shows measurable signs of the beginning of kidney failure, called *azotaemia*. If neglect of the disease continues, your kidneys may fail entirely.

Not every person with diabetes is at equal risk of kidney disease and kidney failure. It seems to be more common in certain families and among certain racial groups, especially Aboriginal Australians, Torres Strait Islanders, South-East Asians, Asian Indians, Chinese and Japanese. It's certainly more common when high blood pressure is present. Although we believe that high blood glucose is the major factor leading to nephropathy, only about 40 per cent of the people who have been poorly controlled go on to develop nephropathy.

Earliest changes

If the kidneys are going to be damaged by diabetic nephropathy, very early on a characteristic finding can be detected in the urine called *microalbuminuria*. A healthy kidney permits only a tiny amount of *albumin*, a protein in the blood, to enter the urine. A kidney that's being damaged by nephropathy is unable to hold back as much albumin, and the level of albumin in the urine increases.

If you've had type 1 diabetes for five years or more or just been diagnosed with type 2 diabetes, your doctor must check for microalbuminuria. If test results are negative, your urine should be checked annually. When microalbuminuria is found, it's still early enough to reverse any damage.

The sophisticated test for microalbuminuria is done by collecting urine over a 24-hour period. However, reliable collections are not always practical, so an easier alternative is to analyse an early-morning specimen of urine. If the level of albumin is abnormally high, it needs to be checked once again to be certain, because some things like exercise can trigger a false positive test.

Macroalbuminuria is diagnosed based on a positive urine test. Once it has been found, the disease can be slowed but not stopped. A second positive test should lead to preventive action to protect the kidneys, and your doctor should devise an appropriate treatment program (see the section 'Getting treatment' later in this chapter).

Doing the simple urine test for microalbuminuria can protect your kidneys from damage. Ask your doctor about it if you think it has never been done. Show this page to your GP if he or she is unclear as to why it's performed.

Progressive changes

After five years of poorly controlled diabetes, significant expansion of the *mesangial tissue*, the cells between the glomeruler capillaries, occurs. The amount of microalbuminuria is very consistent with the amount of mesangial expansion.

Over the next 15 to 20 years, the open capillaries and tubules are squeezed shut by the encroaching tissues and appear like round nodules (known as *Kimmelstiel-Wilson nodules*, after the names of their discoverers). These nodules are diagnostic of diabetic nephropathy. As the glomeruli are replaced by nodules, less and less filtration of the blood can take place. The blood urea nitrogen begins to rise, ultimately ending in *uraemia* when the kidneys aren't doing any cleansing.

Other factors that contribute to the continuing destruction of the kidneys include

- **Abnormal blood fats**, because research shows that elevated levels of certain cholesterol-containing fats promote enlargement of the mesangium.

- **Cigarette smoking**, because heart disease is greatly increased in diabetic nephropathy. Cigarettes are clearly linked to increased occurrence of heart disease.

- **Factors of inheritance**, because certain families and ethnic groups have a higher incidence of diabetic nephropathy.

- **High blood pressure**, which may be almost as important as the glucose level. If the blood pressure is controlled by drugs, the damage to the kidneys slows very significantly. The effect of high blood pressure on the kidneys is shown by the occasional case where a person with diabetes has high blood pressure but also has disease of one of the arteries to a kidney, so that this kidney doesn't feel the force of the blood pressure. While the other kidney goes on to develop nephropathy, this kidney is protected and doesn't develop it.

Diabetic nephropathy doesn't occur alone. Other complications develop at a faster or slower rate. They include

- **Diabetic eye disease:** At the time of complete failure of the kidneys, called *end stage renal disease*, diabetic retinopathy (eye disease) is usually present (see the section 'Having a Look at Eye Disease' later in this chapter). As kidney disease gets worse, retinopathy accelerates. Usually people with retinopathy also have nephropathy. Once proteinuria is present, most patients will also have some retinopathy.

Therefore, if you have diabetes and have proteinuria and retinopathy isn't present, your doctor should look for another cause of kidney disease besides diabetes.

✔ **Diabetic nerve disease, or neuropathy:** Less of an association exists between nephropathy and neuropathy. *Neuropathy* gets worse as kidney disease gets worse, but once dialysis is started, some of the neuropathy disappears, so that part of the neuropathy may be due to wastes that are retained because of the failing kidney rather than true damage to the nervous system. (For more on this condition, see the section 'Reining in Neuropathy, or Nerve Disease' later in this chapter.)

✔ **High blood pressure:** High blood pressure plays an important role in accelerating kidney damage. As kidney failure develops, two-thirds of patients have high blood pressure. With end stage renal disease, almost all have high blood pressure.

✔ **Oedema:** Oedema, or water accumulation, in the feet and legs occurs as the amount of protein in the urine exceeds one or two grams a day.

Getting treatment

Happily, you can avoid all the inconvenience and discomfort associated with diabetic nephropathy.

The following are a few key treatments that your doctor can prescribe to prevent the disease or significantly slow it down once it begins:

✔ **Control your blood glucose:** Tightly controlling your blood glucose helps to reverse the damaging process; such control has been shown to prevent the onset of nephropathy and slow it down once it starts. Both the Diabetes Control and Complications Trial in the United States, which studied glucose control in type 1 diabetes, and the United Kingdom Prospective Diabetes Study Groups in type 2 diabetes have shown this clearly. If you keep your blood glucose close to normal, you will not develop diabetic nephropathy. (For information on controlling your blood glucose, see Part III.)

✔ **Control your blood pressure:** Good control of your blood pressure protects your kidneys from rapid deterioration. Treatment begins with a low-salt diet, but drugs are usually needed. High blood pressure can be controlled by a variety of drugs, but two classes of drug seem particularly valuable in nephropathy. They're called the *angiotensin converting enzyme inhibitors*, or ACE inhibitors, and the *angiotensin receptor blockers*. (See Chapter 10 for more information on ACE inhibitors and angiotensin receptor blockers.)

✔ **Control the blood fats:** Because abnormalities of blood fats seem to make kidney disease worse, it's important to lower the bad, or LDL, cholesterol and raise the good, or HDL, cholesterol while lowering the other fat that's damaging, namely, the triglycerides (refer to the section 'Tracking Cholesterol and Other Fats' later in this chapter). A number of excellent drugs can do this (see Chapter 10).

ACE inhibitors also seem to help the levels of fats. After you've been on an ACE inhibitor for some months, you can take the urine test again to check for a negative result.

✔ **Avoid other damage to the kidneys:** People with diabetes tend to suffer from urinary tract infections, which damage the kidneys. Urinary tract infections must be detected and treated. However, some medications for these infections, such as non-steroidal anti-inflammatory agents (NSAIDS), can damage the kidneys, so these should be avoided. People with diabetes can also have nerve damage to the nerves that control the bladder, producing a neurogenic bladder. (See the section 'Disorders of automatic (autonomic) nerves' later in this chapter.) When the nerves that detect a full bladder fail, proper emptying of the bladder is inhibited and can lead to infections. Intravenous dyes (or contrast) used in some X-ray procedures or angiograms can also damage the kidneys and special precautions may need to be taken if you need to have one of these tests.

✔ **Conduct dialysis if preventive treatment fails:** If dialysis is done, two techniques are currently in use: *Haemodialysis* and *peritoneal dialysis.*

- **Haemodialysis:** The patient's artery is hooked into a tube that runs through a filtering machine that cleanses the blood and then sends it back into the patient's bloodstream. When the patient is moderately well, haemodialysis is done three times a week in a hospital-like setting. However, many complications can potentially develop, including low blood pressure, clotting of the artery and so on. Medication requirements may change when dialysis starts.

- **Peritoneal dialysis:** This technique consists of the insertion of a tube into the body cavity that contains the stomach, liver and intestines, called the *peritoneal cavity.* A large quantity of fluid is dripped into the cavity, and it draws out the wastes, which are then removed as the fluid drains out of the cavity. Peritoneal dialysis is done at home, often on a daily basis. Peritoneal dialysis requires the use of sugar in the fluid so people with diabetes may have very high blood glucose levels unless insulin is added to the bags of dialysis fluid. Once again, this may necessitate a change in diabetes treatment.

Little difference exists in the long-term survival of patients treated with haemodialysis compared with peritoneal dialysis, so the choice becomes one of convenience. People with diabetes don't tolerate kidney failure well, so dialysis tends to be done earlier in them than in people without diabetes.

✔ **Receive a kidney transplant if preventive treatment fails:** Patients who receive a kidney transplant do seem to do better than dialysis patients. Because of a lack of kidneys in Australia, the majority of patients have dialysis rather than a transplant. The transplanted organs are foreign to people who receive them and their bodies try to reject them. Such rejection requires the use of anti-rejection drugs, some of which make diabetic control more complicated. A kidney from a donor who is closely related to the patient is less likely to be rejected. Once a healthy kidney enters the body of a person with diabetes, it's subject to the damage done by elevated glucose levels, so control of the glucose becomes even more important.

Having a Look at Eye Disease

The eyes are the second major organ of the body affected by diabetes over the long term. While some eye diseases, such as glaucoma and cataracts, also occur in people without diabetes, they appear at a higher rate and earlier in people with diabetes. Glaucoma and cataracts respond to treatment very well. Diabetic retinopathy, however, is limited to those with diabetes and may lead to blindness. In the past, blindness was inevitable, but this outcome is far from the case today.

Figure 7-2 illustrates the different parts of the eye.

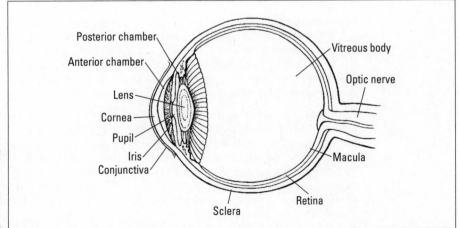

Figure 7-2:
The structure of the eye.

Light enters the eye through the lens, where it's bent and focused upon the retina. The place in the retina where the lens focuses is called the macula. The retina collects an image and transfers it to the optic nerve, which carries it to the brain where the image is interpreted. Between the lens and the retina is a transparent material called the *vitreous body*. (While the eye has many more structures, you don't need to know any more for the purposes of this chapter.)

The eye muscles surround the eye on all sides and are attached to it. These muscles permit you to look up, down and sideways without moving your head. Eye muscles are important in the discussion of diabetic nerve damage, called neuropathy. (For more on this condition, see the section 'Reining in Neuropathy, or Nerve Disease' later in this chapter.)

Recognising common eye diseases

The following eye diseases are commonly found in people with diabetes:

- ✔ **Cataracts:** Cataracts are opaque areas of the lens that can block vision if they're large enough. Cataracts tend to be more common in people with diabetes, even at a young age, both as a result of advanced glycated end products, which form within the lens, and as a result of the increased concentration of sorbitol in the lens. Cataracts can be surgically removed by a fairly routine operation. The entire lens is removed, and an artificial lens is put in its place. With removal, you have an excellent chance for the restoration of your vision.

- ✔ **Glaucoma:** High pressure inside the eye is enough to do damage to the optic nerve. Glaucoma is found more often in people with diabetes than in those without diabetes. If unchecked, the high pressure can destroy the optic nerve and vision along with it. Fortunately, medical treatment can lower the eye pressure and save the eye. Optometrists and eye doctors check for glaucoma on a routine basis.

- ✔ **Retinopathy:** Diabetic retinopathy refers to a number of changes that are seen on the retina of the eye. These changes indicate that the patient has been exposed to high levels of blood glucose over time. If untreated at the appropriate time, retinopathy can lead to blindness. The first changes can be seen after five years of diabetes in both type 1 and 2. Because retinopathy is much more complicated and less treatable than the other two conditions, we discuss it in much more detail later in this chapter.

Checking for eye problems

You must get an annual eye examination by an optometrist or ophthalmologist (a specialist eye doctor) to preserve your vision. All kinds of procedures can be done if abnormalities are found, but they must be discovered first. Get an eye examination as soon as you are diagnosed with type 2 diabetes or five years after being diagnosed with type 1 diabetes, and every year after that.

For the eye examination, the optometrist or ophthalmologist instils drops into your eyes and uses various instruments to examine the pressure, the appearance of your lens and, most importantly, the retina of your eye. Photographs of your retina may be taken. If you see an optometrist and she detects a problem, you may be referred to an ophthalmologist.

You should get your eyes tested annually. Ask if your optometrist or ophthalmologist can send you an automatic reminder each year for your next appointment.

Exploring retinopathy

Ophthalmologists break down retinopathy into two major types, according to their potential to cause visual loss:

- **Background retinopathy:** This type of retinopathy is usually benign but can be a predictor of worse problems. The first changes noted by the ophthalmologist are *retinal aneurysms*, which are the result of weakening of the capillaries of the eye with production of outpocketing of the capillaries. These aneurysms appear as small red dots on the back of the eye. They are benign and disappear over time. The weakened capillaries also rupture sometimes and release blood to form *retinal haemorrhages* and *hard exudates*. The hard exudates, which are yellowish and appear round and sharp, are scars from the haemorrhage. If they extend into the macular area (maculopathy), they reduce vision. If the capillaries in the retina allow fluid and other things to flow into the macula, you get macular oedema and again loss of vision. These exudates and haemorrhages can last for years. As the capillaries close, you have a decreased blood supply to the retina, and *cotton wool spots* or *soft exudates* appear. These represent destruction of the nerve fibre layer because of the lack of blood.

  These changes usually don't cause loss of vision, but in roughly 50 per cent of cases they develop into the more serious proliferative retinopathy.

✔ **Proliferative retinopathy:** This type of retinopathy ends in loss of vision if untreated. Just as in many other parts of the body when the blood supply is reduced, new blood vessels form to carry more blood to the retina. When this happens, the patient is entering the stage of proliferative retinopathy. This is where some visual loss becomes more certain. The growth of blood vessels takes place into the vitreous body. Haemorrhage into the vitreous body blocks vision. As the haemorrhage forms a clot and contracts, it may pull up the retina to produce *retinal detachment*. Because the lens can no longer focus the light on to the macula, you have a complete loss of vision.

Retinopathy, like nephropathy, has a number of important associations:

✔ Certain ethnic groups are at very high risk for retinopathy. These include Aboriginal Australian and Torres Strait Islander populations.

✔ Specific genetic material, if found in a person with diabetes, increases the incidence of retinopathy. At the present time in Australia, DNA testing for predisposition to retinopathy is not routinely done.

✔ Males and females get retinopathy equally.

✔ Greater duration of diabetes results in more eye disease.

✔ High blood pressure worsens the eye disease.

✔ Nephropathy occurs along with the eye disease.

✔ Smoking and alcohol use probably worsen retinopathy (but the final word on this is not in).

✔ Patients with severe diabetic retinopathy are at increased risk for heart attacks.

While no drugs are currently available to treat retinopathy, laser surgery is an excellent treatment option and you can be treated as an outpatient. Laser surgery is used to create a number of burns in the retina and has been shown to save many people's sight. Because the retina is being burned, you have some minor loss of vision. You also have a mild decrease in night vision and a minor decrease in the size of the field that your eye can take in at one time. Laser surgery is also used to successfully treat macular oedema.

Laser surgery is rarely able to treat a retinal detachment that has already occurred. Other surgical procedures, such as a *pneumatic retinopexy*, where a bubble is inserted into the eye and then positioned to help with reattachment of the retina, can be done under local anaesthetic and is successful approximately 80 per cent of the time. If unsuccessful, an operation called a *vitrectomy* may be performed under general anaesthesia. Vitrectomy is successful in restoring some vision about 80 to 90 per cent of the time. If a retinal detachment is also present, the amount of improvement depends upon the extent and duration of the detachment, with restoration of vision occurring about 50 to 60 per cent of the time.

Locating resources for the blind and visually impaired

A search for resources for the blind and visually impaired must begin online. Using a search engine, you can find a huge number of Australian-based sites — and even more worldwide — that have something to do with loss of vision and blindness.

Blind Citizens of Australia (www.bca.org.au) and the Vision Australia Foundation (www.visionaustralia.org.au) provide two of the best Australian sites. (See Chapter 24 for more details on these sites.)

Reining in Neuropathy, or Nerve Disease

The third major organ system of the body that is attacked by poorly controlled diabetes is the nervous system. Forty per cent of people with diabetes have some abnormality of the nervous system but usually don't realise it because this condition doesn't have any early symptoms. These people usually have poor glucose control, smoke and are over 40 years of age. Nerve disease is found most often in those who have had diabetes the longest. The major problem with respect to diabetic neuropathy is the high incidence of foot infections, foot ulcerations and amputations — complications that are all entirely preventable. (See Chapter 8 for more on taking care of your feet.)

How high glucose levels damage nerves remains uncertain. What is found is that the part of the nerve, called the *axon*, that connects to other nerves, or to muscle, degenerates. Researchers believe that the damage is due to a cut-off in the blood supply to the nerve (vascular) in some cases, and to chemical toxins produced by the metabolism of too much glucose (metabolic) in others.

Diabetic neuropathy occurs in any situation where the blood glucose is abnormally elevated for extended periods of time. It is, therefore, not limited to type 1 or type 2 diabetes, although these are the most common diseases where it is found. When the elevated blood glucose is brought down to normal, the signs and symptoms improve. In some cases, the neuropathy disappears.

The fact that intensive control of the blood glucose improves the neuropathy suggests that it's a consequence of abnormal metabolism that damages the nerves.

Diagnosing neuropathy

The speed with which a nervous impulse travels down a nerve fibre is called the *nerve conduction velocity*. In diabetic neuropathy, the nerve conduction velocity (NCV) is slowed. In addition to persistently high blood glucose levels, neuropathy is made worse in the following circumstances:

- **Age:** Neuropathy is most common over the age of 40.

- **Alcohol consumption:** Even small quantities of alcohol can make neuropathy worse.

- **Height:** Neuropathy is more common in taller individuals, who have longer nerve fibres to damage.

Doctors can test nerve function in a variety of ways because different nerve fibres seem to be responsible for different kinds of sensation, such as light touch, temperature and vibration. The connection between the kind of test and the fibre it tests for is as follows:

- **Light touch testing**, perhaps the most important test performed, tests the large fibres, which sense anything touching our skin. This test is done using a monofilament that looks like a hair. The thickness of the filament determines how much force is needed to bend the filament so that it's felt. For example, a monofilament that bends with 1 gram of force can be felt by normal feet. If a patient can feel a monofilament that bends with 10 grams of force, it's unlikely that this person will suffer damage to the foot without feeling it.

   The 10-gram filament can be used by your doctor to discover whether you are at risk of damage to your feet because you cannot feel the pain. This test takes a minute to do and can save your feet from amputation. (See Chapter 8 for more.)

- **Temperature testing**, using a warm or cold item, tests for damage to small fibres, which are very important in diabetes. When small fibres are damaged, people can lose the ability to feel the burn if they inadvertently step into a scalding hot bath.

- **Vibration testing**, using a tuning fork or a machine called a *biothesiometer*, for example, can bring out abnormalities of large nerve fibres.

Symptoms of neuropathy

The various disorders of the nervous system are broken down into the following categories:

✔ **Disorders associated with loss of sensation,** where the sensory nerves are damaged

✔ **Disorders due to loss of automatic (known as *autonomic*) nerves,** which control muscles we don't have to think about, such as the heart muscles, the intestinal muscles and the bladder muscles

✔ **Disorders due to loss of motor nerves,** which carry the impulses to muscles to make them move

The following sections describe the various conditions associated with these disorders.

Disorders of sensation

Disorders of sensation are the most common and bothersome disorders of nerves in diabetes. There are a number of different conditions, which break down into *diffuse neuropathies*, nerve disease where many nerves are involved, and *focal neuropathies*, nerve disease where one or several nerves are involved. This section is about the diffuse neuropathies affecting sensation.

Peripheral neuropathy

Peripheral neuropathy is the most frequent form of diabetic neuropathy. *Peripheral* means on the edge of the body — meaning the feet and hands — and *neuropathy* means disease in the nerves. So, this is a disease of the nerves, presenting itself in the feet and hands. Doctors believe that peripheral neuropathy is a metabolic disease.

The signs and symptoms of peripheral neuropathy are:

✔ Diminished ability to feel light touch or feel the position of a foot, whether bent back or forward, resulting from the loss of the large fibres

✔ Diminished ability to feel pain and temperature from loss of small fibres

✔ Extreme sensitivity to touch

✔ Insignificant weakness

✔ Loss of balance or coordination

✔ Tingling and burning

✔ Worsening of symptoms at night

The danger of this kind of neuropathy is that people don't know, without looking down, whether they have trauma to their feet, such as a burn or an injury from stepping on a piece of glass. When the small nerve fibres are lost, the symptoms are uncomfortable but not as serious. People may feel pain or other uncomfortable sensations especially at night. Treatments are available, but are not always successful in treating the pain. Discuss with your doctor if you have any pain, burning or tingling in your feet.

The most serious complication of loss of sensation in the feet is the neuropathic foot ulcer. Normally, when pressure is applied to a part of the foot, it is felt because of the pain. However, in diabetic neuropathy, this pressure isn't felt. A callus forms and, with continued pressure, the callus softens and liquefies, finally falling off to leave an ulcer. This ulcer may become infected. If it isn't promptly treated, infection can spread. Loss of blood supply to the feet is not an important contributing factor to this type of ulceration — in fact, the blood supply may be very good.

A less common complication in peripheral neuropathy is neuropathic joint damage, or *Charcot's Arthropathy*. In this condition, trauma, which isn't felt, occurs to the joints of the foot or ankle. The bones in the foot get out of line, and many painless fractures may occur. See Chapter 8 for more information on this condition.

Treatment of peripheral neuropathy starts with the best glucose control possible and extremely good foot care. The complications of loss of sensation are preventable. (See Chapter 8 for more on caring for your feet.)

Where pain or other discomfort can be felt, drugs, such as the antidepressants amitriptyline (for example, Tryptanol) or duloxetine (for example, Cymbalta), can reduce these symptoms. A drug called capsaicin (for example, Zostrix cream), which is applied to the skin, reduces pain as well. The results of these treatments are variable and seem to work about 60 per cent of the time. However, the longer the discomfort has been present and the worse it is, the less likely it is that these drugs will work.

If these drugs don't work, other medications may be tried either alone or in combination with the antidepressant drugs. Gabapentin and pregabalin have been found to work more often than many of the older drugs. However, gabapentin and pregabalin do have some side effects, namely sleepiness, dizziness, loss of balance and fatigue, which may make treatment more complicated.

Gabapentin (called Neurontin by the company) has been shown to significantly reduce the discomfort of diabetic neuropathy. Pregabalin (known as Lyrica) has also been found to be effective in some patients with painful diabetic peripheral neuropathy. Patients trialling both drugs were able to sleep better (because diabetic neuropathy is often worse at night). The drugs may work as soon as two weeks after starting treatment, and most patients will have a reduction in painful symptoms with time — although it may take up to 24 months and numbness will remain. However, not all people get a benefit from these treatments.

Diabetic amyotrophy

Diabetic amyotrophy is a mixture of pain and loss of muscle strength in the muscles of the upper leg so that the person can't straighten the knee, and pain extends down from the hip to the thigh. This condition is second in occurrence after peripheral neuropathy. Diabetic amyotrophy generally has a short course but may continue for years and doesn't particularly improve with better diabetic control.

Radiculopathy-nerve root involvement

Sometimes a severe pain in a particular area suggests that the root of the nerve, as it leaves the spinal column, is damaged. The pain is distributed in a horizontal line around one side of the chest or abdomen, and can be so severe that it's mistaken for an internal abdominal emergency. Fortunately, the pain goes away after a variable period of time — usually anywhere from 6 to 24 months.

Disorders of automatic (autonomic) nerves

Many muscle movements are going on all the time, but you're unaware of them. The heart muscle is squeezing down and relaxing. The diaphragm is rising up to empty the lungs of air and relaxing to draw air in. The oesophagus is carrying food down to the stomach from the mouth where, in turn, the stomach pushes it into the small intestine, which pushes it into the large intestine. All these functions of muscles are under the control of nerves from the brain, and diabetic neuropathy can affect them all. These automatic functions are reliant on the autonomic nerves. Depending upon the nerve involved, disorders of the autonomic nerves include:

- ✔ **Bladder abnormalities, starting with a loss of the sensation of bladder fullness.** The urine is not eliminated, and urinary tract infections result. After a while, loss of bladder contraction occurs, and the person has to strain to urinate or loses urine by dribbling. The doctor can easily diagnose this abnormality by finding out how much urine is left in the bladder after urinating. The treatment is to remember to urinate every four hours or take a drug that increases the force of bladder contraction.

- ✔ **Sexual dysfunction in 50 per cent of males with diabetes and 30 per cent of females with diabetes.** Males cannot sustain an erection, and females have trouble lubricating the vagina for intercourse (see the section 'Sexual Problems in Diabetes' later in this chapter for more information on these problems).

- ✔ **Intestinal abnormalities of various kinds.** The most common abnormality is constipation. If nerves to the stomach are involved, the stomach doesn't empty on time. This can lead to 'brittle' diabetes because the insulin is active when no food is available. Fortunately, a drug called metoclopramide helps to empty the stomach. Domperidone has also been found to be helpful in some people if they don't show improvement with metoclopramide.

- ✔ **Involvement of the large intestine that can result in diabetic diarrhoea with as many as ten or more bowel movements in a day.** Accidental loss of bowel contents can occur, and bacteria can grow abnormally in the intestine. This problem responds to antibiotic treatment. Diarrhoea is treated with one of several drugs, which quiets the large intestine.

- ✔ **Heart abnormalities from loss of nerves to the heart.** The heart may not respond to exercise by speeding up as it should. The force of the heart may not increase when the person stands, and the person then becomes lightheaded. A fast fixed heart rate also may occur, and the rhythm of the heart may not be normal. Such people are at risk of sudden death.

- ✔ **Sweating problems, especially in the feet.** The body may try to compensate for the lack of sweating in the feet by sweating excessively on the face or trunk. Heavy sweating can occur when certain foods, such as cheese, are eaten.

- ✔ **Abnormalities of the pupil of the eye.** The pupil determines the amount of light that is let in. As a result of the neuropathy, the pupil is small and doesn't open up in a dark room.

You can see that you can run into all kinds of problems if you develop diabetic neuropathy. None of them need ever bother you, though, if you follow the recommendations in Part III.

Disorders of movement

Neuropathy can affect nerves to various muscles. The result is a sudden inability to move or use those muscles. Researchers believe that these disorders originate as a result of sudden closing of a blood vessel supplying the nerve. The clinical picture depends on which nerve or nerves are affected. If one of the nerves to the eyeball is damaged, the patient cannot turn his eye to the side that nerve is on. If the nerve to the face is affected, the eyelid may droop or the smile on one side of the face may be flat. The patient can have trouble with vision or problems with hearing. Focusing the eye may not be possible. No treatment really exists, but fortunately the disorder goes away of its own accord after several months.

Fighting Heart Disease

In the last three decades, the number of deaths due to heart disease has fallen dramatically, thanks to all kinds of new treatments. Unfortunately, a tremendous increase in the number of type 2 patients is predicted for the next few decades, which may reverse this trend. In this section, you find out about the special problems that diabetes brings to the heart.

Risks of heart disease to people with diabetes

Coronary artery disease (ischaemic heart disease) is the term for the progressive closure of the arteries that supply blood to the heart muscle (atherosclerosis). When one or more of your arteries closes completely, the result is a heart attack (myocardial infarction). In diabetes, the incidence of coronary artery disease (CAD) is increased even in young people with type 1 diabetes. The duration of time with the diabetes is what promotes CAD in type 1 people. No difference occurs in the way CAD affects males or females.

CAD is the most common reason for death in people with type 2 diabetes. Many risk factors promote CAD in the type 2 person, including the following:

✔ **Abnormal blood fats**, especially reduced HDL and increased triglyceride. The abnormal fats may persist even when the glucose is controlled. People without diabetes but with impaired glucose tolerance may show the same abnormalities.

✔ **Central adiposity**, which refers to the distribution of fat particularly in the waist area.

✔ **Hypertension** (high blood pressure).

✔ **Obesity**, often due to lack of exercise and a high-fat diet.

In addition to the known risk factors, there are unknown cardiovascular risk factors related to insulin resistance itself. People with diabetes have more CAD than people without diabetes. When X-ray studies of the heart blood vessels are compared, people with diabetes have more arteries involved than people without diabetes.

If a heart attack occurs, the risk of death is much greater for the person with diabetes. Fifty per cent of people with diabetes die from coronary heart disease compared to 23 per cent of the population without diabetes. The death rate is worse for the person with diabetes who was in poor glucose control before the heart attack. The same poorly controlled person has more complications, such as heart failure, from a heart attack than the person without diabetes. Once a heart attack occurs, the outlook is much worse for the person with diabetes. The death rate five years after the heart attack is 50 per cent, compared with 25 per cent in people without diabetes.

The picture is not a pretty one for the person with diabetes who has coronary artery disease. The treatment options are the same for people with or without diabetes. Treatment to dissolve the clot of blood obstructing the coronary artery can be used, but people with diabetes don't do as well with *angioplasty*, the technique by which a tube is placed into the artery to clean it out and open it up.

People with diabetes do as well with surgery to bypass the obstruction (called *bypass surgery*) as do people without diabetes, but the long-term prognosis for keeping the graft open is not as good.

Metabolic syndrome

The earliest abnormality in type 2 diabetes is insulin resistance, known as metabolic syndrome, syndrome X or insulin resistance syndrome. This syndrome is found in people even before diabetes can be diagnosed. Those with impaired glucose tolerance and even 25 per cent of the population with normal glucose tolerance have evidence of insulin resistance. Several features, all associated with an increased incidence of coronary artery disease, accompany insulin resistance:

- ✔ **Abnormalities of blood fats:** The level of triglycerides is elevated as is the amount of small, dense LDL (*low density lipoprotein*), a particle in the blood that carries cholesterol called 'bad cholesterol'. At the same time, you see a decline in the amount of HDL (*high density lipoprotein*), the 'good' cholesterol particle that helps to clean out the arteries.

- ✔ **Hypertension:** This condition may be a consequence of the increased insulin required to keep the glucose normal when insulin resistance is evident.

- ✔ **Increased abdominal visceral fat:** You can lose a lot of this fat, which is found at the waistline, by dieting and exercising and losing 5 to 10 per cent of your body weight.

- ✔ **Increased plasminogen activator inhibitor-1:** This chemical prevents the breakdown of blood clots that form in the arteries of the heart and other areas.

- ✔ **Obesity:** This is often present in the metabolic syndrome but doesn't need to be present to make the diagnosis.

- ✔ **Sedentary lifestyle:** This is also often the case; however, an active lifestyle doesn't preclude the metabolic syndrome.

The preceding features, plus other features not listed, are found in people who have an increased tendency to suffer coronary artery disease and heart attacks. Keep in mind that the condition is present even when diabetes is not. The condition is probably a primary abnormality and not a consequence of elevated blood glucose over time. When insulin resistance is present in diabetes, the lowering of the blood glucose may decrease the complications of a heart attack, which are related to the high blood glucose, but not the increased tendency to have a heart attack in the first place, which isn't dependent on high blood glucose.

A number of treatments are available for metabolic syndrome. If you're obese and have a sedentary lifestyle, you should correct these problems. It doesn't take a lot of weight loss or exercise to make a major contribution towards decreasing the risk of a heart attack.

You can treat the elevated triglyceride and the reduced HDL with drugs such as the statins or gemfibrozil. Treatment with metformin has also been shown to improve insulin resistance and reduce cardiovascular mortality in people with type 2 diabetes.

Cardiac autonomic neuropathy

Basically, the heart is under the control of nerves, and high glucose levels can damage these nerves. There are a number of ways to test for cardiac autonomic neuropathy:

- **Measure the resting heart rate:** The resting heart rate may be abnormally high (greater than 100).

- **Measure the standing blood pressure:** Blood pressure may fall abnormally low (a decrease of 20 mm Hg sustained for three minutes).

- **Measure the variation in heart rate:** If the variation in heart rate between when you breathe in and when you breathe out is measured, it may be found to be abnormally low (under 10).

The presence of cardiac autonomic neuropathy results in a diminished survival even when there is no coronary artery disease.

Cardiomyopathy

Cardiomyopathy refers to an enlarged heart and scarring of the heart muscle in the absence of coronary artery disease. The heart doesn't pump enough blood with each stroke. The person may be able to compensate with a more rapid heart rate, but if hypertension is present, a stable condition can deteriorate.

The key treatment in this condition is control of the blood pressure as well as control of the blood glucose. Studies in animals in which diabetic cardiomyopathy is induced have shown healing with control of the blood glucose.

Tracking Cholesterol and Other Fats

These days most people are aware of their cholesterol levels — actually, what they know is the level of their *total* cholesterol. Cholesterol circulates in the blood in small packages called *lipoproteins*. These tiny round particles contain fat (*lipo*, as in liposuction) and protein. Because cholesterol doesn't dissolve in water, it would separate from the blood if it weren't surrounded by the protein, just like oil separates from vinegar in salad dressing.

A second kind of fat found in the lipoproteins is *triglyceride*. Triglyceride actually represents the form of most of the fat you eat each day. Although you probably eat only a gram or less of cholesterol (an egg yolk is one-third of a gram of cholesterol), you eat up to 100 grams of triglyceride per day. (For more on the place of fats in your diet, see Chapter 11.) The fat in animal meats is mostly triglycerides.

 When you have your cholesterol checked, find out which particle the cholesterol comes from so that you know whether you have too much bad cholesterol (LDL) or a satisfactory level of good cholesterol (HDL).

Studies show that the risk for coronary artery disease goes up as the LDL cholesterol rises and the HDL cholesterol falls. A study of thousands of people from Framingham, Massachusetts, in the United States, showed that you can get a good picture of the risk by dividing the total cholesterol by the HDL cholesterol. If this result is less than 4.5, the risk is lower. If it's more than 4.5, you're at higher risk of coronary artery disease — and the higher it is, the greater the risk.

The Australian National Heart Foundation deems people with diabetes to be a high-risk group for coronary heart disease. Table 7-1 shows the Heart Foundation's recommended target fat values for people with diabetes.

Table 7-1	Target Fat Levels for People with Diabetes			
	Total Cholesterol	*Triglycerides*	*HDL*	*LDL*
Fasting plasma concentration (mmol/L)	<4	<2	≥1	<2.5

In considering the best treatment for you as regards fat levels, you have to consider other risk factors. You're at:

✔ Highest risk if you already have coronary artery disease, stroke or peripheral vascular disease.

✔ High risk if you

- Are a male over 45

- Are a female over 55

- Smoke cigarettes

- Have high blood pressure

- Have HDL cholesterol less than 1 mmol/L

- Have a father or brother who had a heart attack before age 55

- Have a mother or sister who had a heart attack before age 65

- Have a body mass index greater than 30

✔ Lower risk if you have none of the preceding risk factors.

The treatment then depends on your risk category and level of LDL cholesterol. If you have already had a myocardial infarction, the target for LDL may be lower (that is, less than 2 mmol/L).

Measuring Blood Pressure

Australia is experiencing an epidemic of high blood pressure (*hypertension*) similar to the epidemic of diabetes. The reasons are the same:

✔ Australians are getting fatter. An Australian study has shown that 60 per cent of Australian adults are either obese or overweight, and a slightly larger proportion of this group is male.

✔ Australians are storing fat in the centre of their bodies, the so-called *abdominal visceral fat*.

✔ The population of Australia is ageing — the fastest-growing segment of the population is over 65 years of age. Of people with diabetes, older people have a higher risk of having hypertension.

✔ Australians are more sedentary than before.

People with diabetes have high blood pressure more often than people without diabetes for many reasons besides the preceding ones. For instance, they

- Are prone to kidney disease
- Have increased sensitivity to salt, a substance that raises blood pressure
- Don't experience the nightly fall in blood pressure that normally occurs in people without diabetes

Normal blood pressure is less than 130/85. (The upper reading is known as the *systolic pressure*, while the lower reading is known as the *diastolic blood pressure*.) For years, the diastolic blood pressure was considered more damaging, and an elevation in that pressure was treated with greater importance than an elevation in the systolic blood pressure. Recent studies have shown that it is the systolic blood pressure, not the diastolic blood pressure, that may be more important.

All the complications of diabetes are made worse by an elevation in blood pressure, especially diabetic kidney disease, but also eye disease, heart disease, nerve disease, peripheral vascular disease and cerebral arterial disease.

The United Kingdom Prospective Diabetes Study, published in late 1998, showed clear evidence of the importance of controlling blood pressure in diabetes. This study found that a lowering of blood pressure by 10 mm Hg systolic and 5 mm Hg diastolic resulted in a 24 per cent reduction in any diabetic complication and a 32 per cent reduction in death related to diabetes. A more recent study (the ADVANCE trial) demonstrated similar results, showing that treatment of high blood pressure in people with type 2 diabetes resulted in a 14 per cent reduction in death and an 18 per cent reduction in death from heart attack.

Hypertension affects 44 per cent of people with diabetes and only 10 per cent of people without diabetes. Controlling the blood pressure is absolutely essential in diabetes. Your blood pressure should be no higher than 140/90; if you have kidney disease it should be even lower.

Your doctor should measure your blood pressure at every visit. Better still, get a blood pressure device and measure it yourself. If you detect an elevation, bring it to the attention of your doctor.

Other Diseases of the Vascular System

The same processes that affect the coronary arteries (refer to the section 'Risks of heart disease to people with diabetes' earlier in this chapter) can affect the arteries to the rest of the body, producing peripheral vascular disease, and the arteries to the brain, producing cerebrovascular disease.

Peripheral vascular disease

Peripheral vascular disease (PVD) occurs much earlier in someone with diabetes than in someone without diabetes, and proceeds more rapidly. The clogging of the arteries results in loss of pulses in the feet so that at the time of diagnosis, 8 per cent of men and women no longer feel a pulse in their feet; after 20 years of diabetes, the percentage rises to 45. People with PVD also have a reduction in life expectancy. When PVD occurs, it's much worse in people with diabetes who have much greater involvement of arteries, just as in the heart.

Many risk factors increase the severity of PVD, a couple of which are unavoidable, as follows:

- ✔ **Age**, because the risk of PVD increases as you age
- ✔ **Genetic factors**, because PVD is more common in some families and certain ethnic groups

Take action now to tackle those risk factors that can be successfully eliminated. You need to address the following:

- ✔ **High glucose**, which you can control
- ✔ **Hypercholesterolaemia (high cholesterol)**, which makes PVD worse
- ✔ **Hypertension**, which you can control with tablets if necessary
- ✔ **Obesity**, which you can control
- ✔ **Smoking**, which studies show clearly leads to early amputation and which you can control

In addition to taking action yourself to control or eliminate some of these factors, you can take advantage of certain drugs. Some drugs help prevent closure of the arteries and loss of blood supply — aspirin, which inhibits clotting, is among the most useful.

Cerebrovascular disease

Cerebrovascular disease (CVD) is disease of the arteries that supply the brain with oxygen and nutrients. The risk factors and approach to treatment for cerebrovascular disease are somewhat similar to those for peripheral vascular disease (see preceding section). However, the symptoms are very different because the clogged arteries in CVD supply the brain. If a temporary reduction in blood supply to the brain occurs, the person suffers from a *transient ischaemic attack*, or TIA. This temporary loss of brain function may present itself as slurring of speech, weakness on one side of the body, or numbness. A TIA may disappear after a few minutes, but it comes back again some hours or days later. If a major artery to the brain completely closes, the person suffers a stroke. Fortunately, stroke victims who get medical assistance soon after a stroke can take advantage of clot-dissolving medications.

People with diabetes are at increased risk for CVD just as they are for PVD, and their experience of CVD tends to be worse than it is for the person without diabetes. People with diabetes can suffer from blockage in many small blood vessels in the brain with loss of intellectual function, which is similar to Alzheimer's disease.

Smoking and diabetes

While smoking has many adverse effects on people who don't have diabetes, these effects have been found to be even worse in people with diabetes. Among other things, smoking

✔ Reduces blood flow in arteries and blocks increased flow when it is needed

✔ Increases pain in the legs and hearts of people with PVD and coronary artery disease

✔ Increases *atheromatous plaques*, which are the changes in arteries in the heart

and other areas like the brain and the legs that precede closing of the blood vessels

✔ Increases clustering of platelets, the blood elements that form a plug or clot that blocks the artery

✔ Increases blood pressure, which also worsens atheromatous plaques

These problems don't even take into account the effects of smoking on the lungs, the bladder and the rest of the body.

As the treatable risk factors for CVD are the same as those for PVD (refer to the preceding section), we would encourage you to make every attempt to reduce these risk factors.

Sexual Problems in Diabetes

Diabetes can cause problems with sexual functioning for both men and women. However, with the proper treatment, you can enjoy a rewarding sex life.

Male sexual problems

If carefully questioned, up to 50 per cent of all males with diabetes will admit to some difficulty with sexual function. This difficulty usually takes the form of *erectile dysfunction,* the inability to have or sustain an erection sufficient for intercourse. Many factors besides diabetes cause this problem, and you should rule them out before blaming diabetes. Some other possibilities include the following:

- Hormonal abnormalities, such as insufficient production of the male hormone testosterone or overproduction of a hormone from the pituitary gland, called *prolactin*

- Injury to the penis

- Medications such as some antihypertensives and antidepressants

- Poor blood supply to the penis due to blockage of the artery by peripheral vascular disease, which can be treated very effectively by microvascular surgery

- *Psychogenic impotence,* an inability to have an erection for psychological rather than physical reasons (see the sidebar 'Psychogenic versus physical impotence')

- Other vascular risk factors including hypertension, obesity, known cardiovascular disease and smoking

After you eliminate all the other possibilities for erectile dysfunction, diabetes is then considered to be the source of the problem. In order for you to understand how diabetes affects an erection, we briefly describe how an erection is normally achieved, before discussing how erectile dysfunction caused by diabetes can be treated.

Psychogenic versus physical impotence

Anxiety, stress, depression and conflict with your partner can all cause psychogenic impotence. This type of impotence differs from *organic* (physical) *impotence* in a few ways. Psychogenic impotence is often specific to a particular sexual partner and usually comes on very suddenly. Erections occur during sleep and in the morning, but not when sexual intercourse with that partner is attempted.

Differentiating physical from psychological impotence may require a few nights in a sleep lab, where a device that detects erections during sleep is placed around the penis. Men without physical impotence normally have three or more erections during sleep, while their eyes are going through a state of rapid eye movement (REM). Doctors can measure both the erections and REM. If erections occur at various times of day or night, the impotence is psychological and not physical.

Psychological impotence is very responsive to counselling, especially if done together with the female partner with whom the problem occurs.

Impeding the erection process

As a result of some form of stimulation, whether by touch, sight, sound or something else, the brain activates nerves in the parasympathetic nervous system (part of the autonomic nervous system). These nerves cause muscles to relax so that blood flow into the penis greatly increases. As blood flow increases, the veins through which blood leaves the penis compress, and the penis becomes erect. When the penis is erect, it contains about 11 times as much blood as when it's flaccid. With sufficient stimulation, muscles contract, propelling semen through the *urethra* (the tube in the penis that normally carries urine from the bladder) to the outside of the body. The pleasant sensation that occurs along with the muscle contractions *(ejaculation)* is called *orgasm*.

Orgasm and ejaculation are the result of stimulation by the other side of the autonomic nervous system, the sympathetic nervous system. As the stimulation causes contraction of the muscles, it closes the muscle over the bladder so that urine doesn't normally accompany expulsion of semen and the semen doesn't go back into the bladder.

Diabetes can damage the parasympathetic nervous system so that the male can't get an erection sufficient for sexual intercourse. The sympathetic nervous system is spared, so that ejaculation and orgasm can occur. Of course, intercourse may be unpleasant for the partners because of the consequences of the inability of the male to achieve a firm erection.

The onset of failure of erection is determined by the following factors:

- ✔ **Degree of control of the blood glucose:** Better control is associated with fewer problems.

- ✔ **Duration of the diabetes:** The longer you have diabetes, the more likely it is that you will be unable to have an erection.

- ✔ **Interaction with the partner:** A positive relationship is important.

- ✔ **State of mind:** A positive attitude with less anxiety is associated with more successful erections.

- ✔ **Use of drugs or alcohol:** Both may prevent erection.

Treating erectile dysfunction

Fortunately for the male with diabetes and with erectile dysfunction, numerous approaches to treatment exist, beginning with drugs, continuing with external devices to create an erection, and ending with implantable devices that provide a very satisfactory erection. Treatment is successful in between 70 and 80 per cent of men, but only a small percentage ever discuss the problem with their doctor.

Treatment options for erectile dysfunction include the following:

- ✔ **Oral tablets such as Viagra, Levitra or Cialis:** These medications belong to the same class of drug called phosphodiesterase inhibitors. They work by relaxing the blood vessels in the penis when a man becomes sexually aroused. These drugs work quickly regardless of age or severity of the condition and its underlying cause. However, these drugs are not free of side effects. Some men experience headaches, light-headedness, dizziness, distorted vision, facial flushing or indigestion. These side effects generally decline with continued use of the drug. The drugs don't seem to affect diabetes control.

  One important group of men must not take drugs such as Viagra. Men who have chest pain often take nitrate drugs, the most common of which is nitroglycerine. The combination of Viagra and nitrates may cause a significant and possibly fatal drop in blood pressure.

- ✔ **Injection into the penis:** You can inject alprostadil (marketed as Caverject) directly into the penis to create an erection. Alprostadil is a chemical that relaxes the blood vessels in the penis to allow more flow, and doesn't require sexual stimulation in order to work. The drug is injected about 30 minutes before intercourse and no more than once in 24 hours and three times per week. An injection of alprostadil gives a full erection lasting about an hour in 85 to 95 per cent of men, except for those who have the most severe loss of blood flow to the penis. Complications of injections are rare but include bruising, pain and the formation of nodules at the injection site.

A very rare complication of injecting alprostadil into the penis is *priapism,* where the penis maintains its erection for many hours. If the erection lasts for more than four hours, you must see your doctor to get an injection of a *vasoconstrictor,* a drug that squeezes down the arteries into the penis so that blood flow is interrupted.

✔ **Vacuum constriction devices:** These tubes, which fit over the penis, create a closed space when pressed against the patient's body. A pump draws out the air in the tube, and blood rushes into the penis to replace the air. Once the penis is erect, a rubber band is placed around the base of the penis to keep the blood inside it. The rubber band may be kept on for up to 30 minutes.

✔ **Implanted penile prostheses:** If Viagra doesn't work and you don't like the idea of injecting yourself in your penis or using a vacuum device, a *prosthesis* (an artificial substitute) can be implanted in the penis to give a very satisfactory erection. These come in several varieties. A semi-rigid type produces a permanent erection, but some men don't like the inconvenience of a permanent erection. An inflatable prosthesis involves a pump in the scrotal sac that contains fluid. The pump can be squeezed to transfer the fluid into balloons in the penis to stiffen it. When not pumped up, the penis appears normally soft. In the past few years, the surgery to insert these prostheses has become very satisfactory.

Female sexual problems

Because the female doesn't have a penis that must enlarge for sex, the sexual complications of diabetes aren't as visually obvious. However, the problems can be just as difficult for women. Because several of these problems are also seen in menopause, particularly the dry vagina and irregular menstrual function, menopause must be ruled out first.

The following problems are associated with diabetes:

✔ You may have a dry mouth and dry vagina because of the high blood glucose.

✔ Your menstrual function may be irregular when your diabetes is out of control.

✔ You may develop yeast infections (such as thrush) of the vagina that make intercourse unpleasant.

✔ Because type 2 diabetes is usually associated with obesity, you may feel fat and unattractive.

- ✔ You may feel uncomfortable discussing the problem with your partner or your doctor.

- ✔ You may have loss of bladder control due to a neurogenic bladder.

- ✔ Your increasing age may result in a reduction in oestrogen secretion and vaginal thinning and dryness.

The female with long-standing diabetes may have several other problems that are specific to her sexual organs. These problems include:

- ✔ **Reduced lubrication because of parasympathetic nerve involvement:** Lubrication serves to permit easier entry of the penis, but it also increases the sensitivity of the vagina to touch, thus increasing pleasant sensations.

- ✔ **Reduced blood flow because of diabetic blood vessel disease:** Some of the lubrication comes from fluid within the blood vessels.

- ✔ **Loss of skin sensation around the vaginal area:** This reduces pleasure.

Most women who have problems with lubrication use over-the-counter preparations to lubricate themselves. These preparations fall into three categories:

- ✔ Oil-based lubricants, like vegetable oils

- ✔ Petroleum-based lubricants, but these are not recommended because of the possibility of bacterial infection

- ✔ Water-based lubricants, like K-Y jelly

The lubrication product you use is a matter of choice, although water-based products are probably the easiest to use and clean up, and the safest if using condoms.

Oestrogen, which can be taken by mouth or placed in the dry vagina in pessary form, also may be useful for the postmenopausal woman. Talk to your GP or gynaecologist about finding the right combination of treatments to suit you.

When psychological or interpersonal issues exist, a discussion with a counsellor, the use of antidepressant medications (although some of these can dry the vagina), and sex counselling with your partner are important steps to take to improve sexual pleasure.

As with all of the problems associated with diabetes that you read about in this book, maximum control of the blood glucose prevents or slows down a lot of these complications.

Skin Disease in Diabetes

Many conditions involve the skin and are unique to the person with diabetes because of the treatment and complications of the disease. The most common complications involving the skin include the following:

- *Acanthosis nigricans*, a velvety-feeling increase in pigmentation on the back of the neck and the armpits, causes no medical problems and needs no specific treatment. This condition is usually found when *hyperinsulinaemia* (excessive amounts of insulin) and insulin resistance are present, and is also seen in children with type 2 diabetes.

- *Alopecia*, or loss of hair, occurs in type 1 diabetes (for unknown reasons).

- Diabetic thick skin, which is thicker than normal skin, occurs in people who have had diabetes for more than ten years. This includes Dupuytren's contractures, where fascia under the skin of the palms can thicken and cause contraction of the skin. This can affect the hand tendons, which can be corrected with surgery.

- Dry skin, which is a consequence of diabetic neuropathy, leading to a lack of sweating.

- Fungal infections occur under the nails or between the toes. Fungus likes moisture and elevated glucose. Lowering the glucose and keeping the toes dry prevents these infections. Medications may cure this problem, but it recurs if glucose and moisture aren't managed.

- *Insulin hypertrophy* (fat hypertrophy) is the accumulation of fatty tissue where insulin is injected. This normal action of insulin is prevented by moving the injection site around.

- *Insulin lipoatrophy* (fat atrophy) is loss of fat where the insulin is injected. Although the cause is unknown, the condition is rarely seen now that human insulin has replaced beef and pork insulin.

- *Necrobiosis lipoidica*, which also affects people without diabetes, creates patches of reddish-brown skin on the shins or ankles; the skin becomes thin and can ulcerate. Females tend to have this condition more often than males. Corticosteroid injections may be used, and the areas eventually become depressed and brown.

- *Vitiligo* (loss of skin pigmentation) is part of the autoimmune aspect of type 1 diabetes and can't be prevented.

- *Xanthelasma*, which are small yellow flat areas called plaques on the eyelids, occur even when cholesterol is not elevated.

Chapter 8

Fabulous Feet

Among the long-term complications for people with diabetes, two that have particular ramifications for the feet of people with diabetes are peripheral neuropathy and peripheral vascular disease (refer to Chapter 7). Because of these conditions, people with diabetes are more prone to a range of foot problems, from numbness, burning and tingling, to ulcers and very occasionally amputation.

The most recent statistics tell us that around 3,400 amputations occur in Australia each year in people with diabetes (that's 65 per day!). People with diabetes have a 15 to 40 per cent increased risk of a lower limb amputation compared with the general population. Despite improved detection and treatment of diabetes-related foot problems, the number of diabetes-related amputations is actually rising. (This may be because we're getting better at classifying foot problems as being related to diabetes, but even so, it's a worrying trend.)

The good news, however, is that diabetic feet can be fabulous, it just takes a little more care — from you and from your diabetes care team. This chapter covers common foot problems and how you can prevent them, assessing your feet for these problems and how you can treat them if they do arise.

Understanding Common Foot Problems

All feet are prone to problems such as bunions, corns and nail deformities, especially if you wear ill-fitting shoes. However, these problems can become much more serious if you have diabetes. In this section, we cover the common problems diabetic feet are prone to.

Dry, cracked skin

People with diabetes are prone to dry, cracked skin as a result of nerve damage. Not only does this feel uncomfortable and itchy, cracks in the skin allow bacteria to get in and cause infection. Scratching the skin causes further cracks and openings in the skin and increases the risk of both bacterial and fungal infection.

Synthetic socks can cause a build-up of moisture in the foot and make dry, cracked skin on your feet worse. Choose socks made out of cotton or natural fibres.

Calluses and corns

High-heeled, long, narrow shoes may look gorgeous but can result in areas of thickened skin at sites of pressure, known as calluses or corns. While anyone will develop thickened skin at pressure points, in a person with diabetes the risks from this condition are much greater because the area becomes a potential site for ulceration.

Calluses and corns require skilful attention from a podiatrist. To avoid them, always wear shoes that fit well and don't squeeze or put pressure on your feet.

See the section 'If the shoe fits — wear it!' later in this chapter for more on the type of shoes you should be wearing — and when you should be wearing them.

Diabetic foot ulcers

Diabetic foot ulcers can be a major problem for people with diabetes, mainly due to a lack of feeling in the feet and poor circulation.

Obviously, if your feet feel numb, you can injure your feet without being aware of it — for example, you could stand on a sharp stone or cut your foot and be totally unaware that you've done so. You could walk around with a pebble in your shoe for a week without feeling it.

A foot ulcer can develop from such a minor injury to the foot — and if you have limited vision or mobility, you may not be able to see the ulcer, allowing it to progress. People with diabetes are also prone to poor circulation and swelling of the feet, which slow down the healing process for foot ulcers. If the ulcer gets infected, the situation gets even worse.

Intact skin acts as an important barrier to infection, so if diabetic foot ulcers are not treated promptly, infection may set in. This infection could involve the bone, making treatment much more difficult and possibly even requiring amputation to control the infection.

The progression from injury to foot ulcer to severe infection may be more rapid in people with poor control of their diabetes.

Identified risk factors for diabetic ulcers include the following:

- Abnormal foot structure
- Being male
- Evidence of peripheral neuropathy (refer to Chapter 7)
- Long duration of diabetes
- Poor circulation
- Previous ulceration
- Smoking

Key components of diabetic ulcer management include the following:

- Antibiotics (where appropriate)
- Avoidance of weight bearing (if the ulcer is on the sole of the foot)
- Establishment of good blood supply
- Regular wound dressings

Ulceration and infection of the foot is best managed by a multidisciplinary specialist team with expert knowledge in endocrinology, orthopaedics, vascular medicine and podiatry.

Foot infections

If you have diabetes, you generally have a higher risk of bacterial or fungal infections. In Australia's mostly hot and often humid climate, fungal infections of the foot and between the toes are common. Bacterial infections may occur more easily if the skin is dry and cracked. Any of these infections can cause more serious complications in people with diabetes, such as ulcers or even amputation.

Foot deformity

Diabetes can also affect motor nerves that supply leg muscles (refer to Chapter 7). Nerve damage can lead to a condition of the toes called 'clawing' and the loss of the arch in the foot. This redistributes the load on the foot, making walking more unbalanced. This unbalanced gait puts excessive pressure on certain parts of the sole of the foot, which can cause ulceration (refer to the section 'Diabetic foot ulcers' earlier in this chapter).

In the most severe cases of damage to the motor nerves, what's known as *Charcot's Arthropathy* (also known as *Charcot's Foot*) may develop, leaving the person at high risk of ulcers on the bottom of the deformed foot and risking fractures of the bones of the foot (which can't be felt). The foot becomes unusable.

Caring for Your Feet — Prevention is Better than Cure

The key to fabulous feet — and successful long-term foot care — is prevention. Stopping problems occurring is a lot easier than trying to correct them down the track. Prevention involves you, and your podiatrist, gaining an intimate knowledge of your feet, and making sure you put your best foot forward — in appropriate footwear!

Checking your feet

So you can identify potential foot problems before they become serious, you should inspect your feet every day, including checking the sole of the foot and between the toes. Look for anything that's abnormal or wasn't present the previous day.

Problems and changes you should be looking for during your daily foot inspection include the following:

- Bleeding
- Blisters
- Bruises
- Calluses
- Changes in colour or temperature
- Cracks in the skin
- Fungal infections
- Ingrown toenails
- Swelling
- Wet soggy skin

If you find it difficult to see under your feet, use a mirror. If you can't see properly, ask someone to look at your feet for you.

If you find a problem, do something about it immediately. For minor injuries such as scratches, wash the area with tap or salty water (not hot) and cover with a non-stick dressing.

If you can see no improvement in a problem area on your foot after 24 to 48 hours, or the wound becomes red and hot, see your GP or podiatrist.

Looking after skin and nails

As well as checking your feet daily for any problems or changes, you want to implement a daily foot care routine. Do the following at least daily:

- **Wash your feet daily in warm water with a mild soap.** Always check the temperature of the water with your elbow first to make sure it's not too hot.

✔ **After washing, dry your feet carefully, particularly the skin between your toes.** If this skin becomes white and soggy, apply a small amount of methylated spirits using a cotton bud.

If you have white, soggy skin between your toes that isn't fixed by applying methylated spirits, see your GP. You may have a fungal infection requiring anti-fungal medication.

✔ **Apply a urea-based moisturising cream.** This helps prevent the skin getting too dry. Apply the cream twice daily.

You also need to be careful about the state of your toenails. If you can cut your own nails, cut them straight across and not too short. Check afterwards to ensure you haven't left any sharp edges; if sharp edges are present, use a nail file to smooth them.

See a podiatrist to cut your nails if

✔ You have problems reaching or seeing your feet

✔ Your nails are thickened or otherwise abnormal

Making friends with your podiatrist

Podiatrists are trained to recognise any serious foot problems that require urgent attention. When you have diabetes, your podiatrist (your new best friend!) can assess your feet and give you unbiased advice on how to choose footwear and look after your feet between visits.

Like any good friend, your podiatrist may give you advice that you don't want to hear (especially concerning appropriate footwear). Your health is more important than fashion, however — and your podiatrist may even be able to give you some tips on where you can buy shoes that are both appropriate and fashionable.

The number of times you should visit your podiatrist per year depends on the condition of your feet and the overall control of your diabetes. If you're independent and can feel your feet, see your feet and reach your feet, you may require only a yearly check-up. If you have calluses or major foot deformities, and have been diagnosed as at very high risk, you may need review every two to three weeks. If you have an ulcer, your visits may be as frequent as every one to two weeks.

The Australian government subsidises a number of visits to a podiatrist per year for people with diabetes. Your GP can organise this.

If the shoe fits — wear it!

Foot ulceration and infection can be devastating to a person with diabetes; however, the good news is that foot ulcers are preventable! Prevention starts with having well-fitted, appropriate footwear, and wearing this footwear all the time — not just to the diabetes clinic or podiatrist. Good shoes aren't cheap, but they're an important investment in your health.

You need to wear shoes at all times — including in the house, at the beach, in the ocean and at the pool, particularly if you have numbness of the feet. Swim booties are suitable for the beach or the pool, but thongs and open shoes aren't appropriate.

When choosing appropriate footwear, look out for the following features:

- Adequate width
- Laces or velcro straps to keep the foot securely in the shoe
- Leather or mesh uppers to allow air to circulate
- Low, firm heel
- Rubber sole at least 5 millimetres thick

Your podiatrist can advise you on choosing appropriate shoes and can assess whether your shoes are right for you. Your podiatrist can also direct you to specialist shops that understand the needs of people with diabetes, which can be found in most larger Australian cities.

Because your feet tend to swell through the day, shop for shoes in the afternoon. Once you've made a purchase, test out your new shoes for about 30 minutes, then take them off and inspect your feet for redness or blistering. Make sure you can return new shoes if they're not suitable.

Always feel inside your shoes before you put them on. A small pebble in a shoe can lead to months of misery. And always wear socks or stockings (made from natural fibres) with your shoes.

Even the best fitting shoes, socks and orthotics wear out! Replace them as needed — particularly if you have foot deformities and so have abnormal distribution of pressure on the soles of your feet.

Booking a Foot Assessment

Soon after you've been diagnosed with type 2 diabetes, see your doctor or podiatrist for an assessment of your feet to check blood supply and nerve function. Any problems with either need to be identified and treated.

If you have type 1 diabetes, a foot assessment at diagnosis is not required as the onset of the diabetes has been short and problems haven't had a chance to arise. However, your doctor should check your feet at every visit and a trip to the podiatrist to learn how to care for your feet is a good investment.

Help from Medicare is available for podiatry treatment for all people with diabetes. Speak with your GP about making the appropriate arrangements.

Your GP or podiatrist assesses the shape of your feet, and searches for any evidence of ulceration or skin thickening and for infections, swelling, dryness and cracks or moist areas (particularly between the toes). A podiatrist also notes the temperature and colour of the feet, any major difference between the two feet, and any change from lying to standing. He or she checks the pulses at your ankle, foot and knees, inspects your footwear and may ask you to take a few steps to assess your gait.

Feeling in your foot is tested with cotton wool, a monofilament, a tuning fork or a machine called a biothesiometer (refer to Chapter 7 for more on testing options).

You also need to provide blood samples so your GP can assess your diabetes control and possibly identify any other factors that may contribute to foot problems (such as vitamin deficiencies). Blood flow can then be further tested using a Doppler machine and an ultrasound probe on the skin.

If any evidence of ulceration or infection is present, further tests may be needed to assess the extent of the problem.

You can help your GP and podiatrist arrive at a better assessment of your feet and general health by providing as much information as possible. Describe all your symptoms, including abnormal feeling, cold feet and discomfort on walking up a hill. Also be honest about your smoking!

Treating Foot Problems

If you are unfortunate enough to suffer foot damage and experience problems with your feet, different treatment options are available depending on the problem that has occurred. Your options can be as straightforward as taking drugs to treat the symptoms of neuropathy or an infection, or they can involve more complex surgical procedures.

Considering medications

Despite your best efforts, problems with your feet may develop that require medication.

The pain associated with peripheral sensory neuropathy (which may include intense tingling in the feet or pins and needles, which often gets worse at night) is sometimes treated with drugs that include amitriptyline (also used as an antidepressant) or gabapentin (also used as an anticonvulsant). As with all medications, risks and benefits exist with these drugs, so remember to ask your GP or diabetes specialist about these.

Bacterial infections may complicate ulcers and require antibiotics. Commonly used oral antibiotics include cephalosporins, anti-staphylococcal penicillins, clindamycin and amoxycilln/clavulanate. Infections involving the bone require higher doses of antibiotics and a prolonged course of treatment; intravenous antibiotics are usually required in this situation.

If your GP or diabetes specialist prescribes antibiotics, you need to complete the whole course, even if you're feeling better.

Fungal infections of the foot and toenails such as tinea are very common for people with diabetes, and these infections often require prolonged topical or oral anti-fungal agents.

Many other disorders can mimic tinea infections of the toenails, and using tinea treatments when something else is the cause of your infection can have serious side-effects. If you have a foot infection, always see your GP to confirm the diagnosis.

Avoiding surgery

Doctors try to avoid surgery if possible, because losing a toe (or more) can be very psychologically distressing, a period of recovery is required and the loss of a toe can change the biomechanics of the foot in such a way that walking becomes more difficult and remaining toes can start to claw.

When you have diabetes, wound healing may be impaired and the risk of infection is higher, so the decision to operate should never be taken lightly.

However, you may require foot surgery for a variety of reasons. Bunions may become painful and interfere with walking and toes may need to be straightened. At times an amputation is the only way to control infection in the foot.

In some cases, the amputation can be quite severe. The operation needs to be extensive enough to ensure all the infection is removed, and sometimes what appears on the surface to be a small area of ulceration can actually be a much more extensive area of disease.

The best way to avoid surgery is preventing foot problems from occurring. Your feet are precious — look after them!

Part III
Living with Diabetes: Your Physical Health

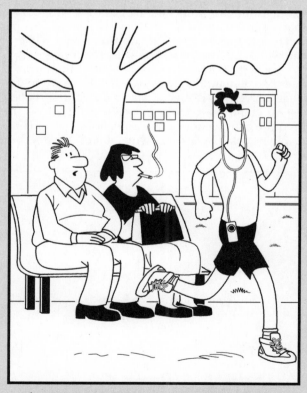

'If Bob has diabetes, how come he looks so much fitter than us?'

In this part . . .

1s it possible that you could be healthier with diabetes than your friends who don't have diabetes? This part shows that the answer to that question is yes. While others without diabetes, who may not be aware they even have any health problems, are left to their own devices, you can find out exactly what you have to do — not just to live with diabetes, but to thrive with diabetes. The steps you need to take are simple and basic — they just require a little effort. In no time, however, you'll probably be asking yourself: 'Why didn't I think of that?'

Chapter 9

Glucose Monitoring and Other Tests

*I*f you read Part II, you know all about the complications that can happen to you if you have diabetes. In the next four chapters (Part III), we now discuss the options you can adopt to help you avoid these complications and manage your diabetes. Things are improving all the time — most of the products and treatments covered in this Part weren't available 20 years ago, and some of the new products now available can have a dramatic effect on how well you manage your diabetes. While you may think it's a bit of an inconvenience and an expense, your health is worth it.

Part II wasn't intended to worry you, but to set out clearly just what having diabetes can involve. In this chapter, you discover all you need to know to put your diabetes in its proper place. You find out how well you're currently controlling your blood glucose and what changes you need to make in your treatment to ensure your target blood glucose levels are met.

Testing, Testing: Tests You Need to Stay Healthy

How are doctors actually doing in medical care for a person with diabetes? In Sydney, staff at the St Vincent's Hospital Diabetes Centre looked at whether standard tests that should be performed regularly on patients with diabetes had been completed. Staff documented whether glycosylated haemoglobin (HbA1c) had been checked, whether an annual dilated eye examination (which can be done by your optometrist) had been completed, whether blood pressure and *lipids* (blood fats) had been measured recently and whether kidney and nerve function had also been reviewed. Staff also checked whether the diabetes educator and dietitian services provided were used appropriately.

The results revealed the following:

- Almost two-thirds of the centre's patients had the majority of these tests completed on a regular basis.

- One-third of the people had seen a diabetes educator and less than one-fifth had seen a dietitian in the previous two years.

- More than half of those with type 1 diabetes were achieving an HbA1c of less than 8 per cent and two-thirds of those with type 2 diabetes were also meeting this target. (See the section 'Tracking Your Glucose over Time with Glycosylated Haemoglobin' for more on target levels.)

- About half of the centre's patients with type 1 diabetes and about one-third of patients with type 2 diabetes were achieving recommended blood pressure goals.

- Half the patients with either type 1 or type 2 diabetes were achieving the targets for blood fats.

Obviously, doctors and members of diabetes care teams can still do more to ensure all patients are tested appropriately and that more people achieve their target health goals; however, these results also reflect a need for the person with diabetes to be more aware of what's required to manage their condition. Knowing what's required means you can monitor your own management of diabetes — and remind your doctors as needed! This chapter provides everything you need to know.

Monitoring Your Blood Glucose

Insulin was extracted and used for the first time more than 80 years ago. Since then, nothing has improved the life of people with diabetes as much as the ability to measure their own blood glucose with a drop of blood. Prior to blood glucose self-monitoring, testing the urine for glucose was the only way to determine whether blood glucose was high, but urine testing couldn't tell at all whether the glucose was low. The urine test for glucose is therefore worthless for controlling blood glucose, although testing the urine for other things such as ketones and protein can be of value.

Understanding the technology is simple enough. The glucose in a drop of your blood reacts with an enzyme on a special test strip. The reaction produces electrons, and a meter (electronic) then converts the amount of electrons into a glucose reading. Each meter (glucometer) has its own corresponding test strip. They aren't interchangeable!

One of the first things that was learnt when blood glucose self-testing became available is that a person with diabetes, even someone whose condition is fairly stable, can have tremendous variation in glucose levels, especially in association with food, but even in the fasting state before breakfast. This is why multiple tests are needed throughout the day.

How often should you test?

How often you test is determined by the kind of diabetes you have, the kind of treatment you're using and the level of stability of your blood glucose levels, as follows:

✔ **If you have type 1 diabetes and you're on four or more insulin injections per day or on an insulin pump, you need to test before each meal and at bedtime.** The reason is that you're constantly using the information you gain to make adjustments to your insulin doses. No matter how good you think your control is, you cannot feel the level of the blood glucose without testing, unless you're hypoglycaemic (and even this can be missed at times). If you try to guess your blood glucose before you test it, no doubt you find that you're close less than 50 per cent of the time. Inaccuracy like this is not sufficient for good glucose control.

Occasionally, people with type 1 diabetes should test two hours after a meal and in the middle of the night to see just how high the glucose goes after eating and whether it's going too low in the middle of the night.

- **If you have type 2 diabetes and are on insulin, you need to test three to four times per day.** Remember to vary the times so you test both before and after meals. Testing at these times will help you to assess whether the treatment and doses you are on are the most appropriate.

- **If you have type 2 diabetes and you're on tablets, you need to test twice per day.** Testing twice per day at varying times helps you measure the effect of the treatment. If your glucose levels are consistently stable — between 4 and 8 mmol/L over several weeks or one month — you may only need to test once per day, alternating between pre- and 2 hours post-meals. Testing in this manner can be enough to keep you aware of your diabetes control.

- **If you have type 2 diabetes and are just on diet and exercise, you don't need to test.** If you're able to manage your diabetes with just diet and exercise, you shouldn't need to frequently monitor your blood glucose levels — but always check what your GP or diabetes educator advises. You still need to have a glycosylated haemoglobin test every four to six months to ensure your glucose levels continue to be stable. (See the section 'Tracking Your Glucose over Time with Glycosylated Haemoglobin' later in this chapter for more on this test.)

- **If you're pregnant, see the testing guidelines outlined in Chapter 18.** Expectant mothers are encouraged to test between six and seven times per day in order to keep their developing foetus as healthy as possible.

Blood glucose testing can be useful in showing you how the things you do through the day affect your blood glucose levels. If you eat something not normally part of your diet and want to test its effect on your glucose, do a test. If you're about to exercise, a blood glucose test can tell you whether you need to eat before starting the exercise or whether you can use the exercise to bring your glucose down. If your diabetes is temporarily unstable and you're about to drive, you can test before getting into the car to make sure that you're not on the verge of hypoglycaemia.

How do you perform the test?

If you don't already have a meter, the next section on choosing one is essential reading. Performing a blood glucose test is quite straightforward — while all blood glucose meters work a little differently, all meters require a drop of blood, usually from the finger. To get a drop of blood, you can use a finger-prick lancet, either on its own or contained within an automatic device. Many automatic devices are spring-loaded so you push a button and the lancet springs out and pricks your finger. Some glucose meters come with their own recommended finger-prick devices.

To perform a blood glucose test, you need the following:

- ✔ Blood glucose meter
- ✔ Blood glucose record book
- ✔ Cotton wool ball or tissue
- ✔ Disposable test strip
- ✔ Lancet device

Your meter will have an in-built memory, so make sure the correct date and time are set on it. That way, you can look back at the reading and know whether it was taken in the early morning or late at night! Some meters allow you to download these readings onto a computer, so you can print out the results and take them with you when you see your doctor or diabetes educator.

Keep a blood glucose record book where you can write down each of your readings, even if your meter has a memory. Writing down the results enables you to reflect on your glucose levels at different times of the day and to see the effect different foods or activities have on your glucose level. You can then discuss these different situations with your doctor, diabetes educator and/or dietitian. Record books are available from your local diabetes centre or the Australian Diabetes Council (in NSW) or Diabetes Australia in other states and territories.

Keep the following in mind when you're testing your glucose:

- ✔ **Wash your hands with soap and warm water and dry thoroughly.**

- ✔ **If you have trouble getting blood, warm up your hand.** Rub your hands together or put them under warm water.

- ✔ **If your meter requires a code, make sure that the code for the strips matches the code in the meter.**

- ✔ **Prepare the lancing device by inserting a fresh lancet.** Lancets that are used more than once are not as sharp as a new lancet, and can cause more pain and injury to the skin.

- ✔ **Discard any unused strips in the vial after 90 days as the test strips may deteriorate.** Studies have shown that the qualities of test strips that are loose in a vial deteriorate rapidly if the vial is left open. Two hours of exposure to air may ruin the strips, so be sure to replace the cap on the vial. Strips that are individually foil-wrapped don't have this problem.

- ✔ **Don't let others use your meter.** The test results of others will be mixed in with your tests if they're downloaded into a computer or if your GP or diabetes care team go back through the meter's memory to see what's been happening.

Light, moisture and heat can all adversely affect the test strips. Ensure the lid is tightly fastened after use, you store the strips in a cool, dry place (not the refrigerator!) and you keep the *desiccant* (usually a small, white packet) in the bottle.

Investigating Blood Glucose Meters

So many meters are on the market that you may be confused about which one to use. One consideration that should play no part in your decision is its cost; some manufacturers are happy to give you the meter because you're required to purchase their test strips. Each manufacturer makes a different test strip, and they're not interchangeable with other machines. The cost of blood glucose meters has dropped dramatically over the years and a reliable meter costs less than $50.

Because the meters are so cheap and the science is changing so rapidly, get a new meter every year or two to make sure that you have the latest state of the art. The cost of test strips is the same from meter to meter, so their cost doesn't have to play a big role in your meter decision, either.

Another aspect that you need not be concerned about is the accuracy of the various machines. All are accurate to a degree acceptable for managing your diabetes. Keep in mind, though, that they don't have the accuracy of a laboratory. They are probably different by about 10 per cent (above or below) compared to what can be achieved in a laboratory.

Choosing the right meter for you

Doctors sometimes have meters that they prefer to work with because a computer program can download the test results from the meter and display them in a certain way. This analysis can be enormously helpful in deciding how to adjust your treatment for the best control of your glucose, but it's not essential.

To satisfy yourself that you have the right meter for your purposes, ask the following questions when choosing a meter:

- Does the manufacturer provide a readily available and reliable back-up service?

- If a meter is manufactured overseas, is servicing for it available in Australia and is the warranty valid here? And are the results produced by the meter measured in mmol/L?

✔ If a small child is to use it, can the child easily use the meter and strips? Some meters are easier to use than others. Some require a tiny sample of blood, meaning a smaller and less painful finger prick is possible.

✔ Are the batteries readily available or are they hard to get and expensive?

✔ Does the meter have a memory that you or your doctor can check?

✔ Is the data stored on the meter downloadable to a computer program that can manipulate the data?

✔ How quickly does the meter display the results? Some meters can display results in as little as five seconds.

✔ Does the meter offer more advanced options? Some meters allow you to enter events (like eating or exercising) and come with software programs that allow you to download data to a computer. This feature is particularly helpful for people who test frequently and use intensive insulin treatment.

✔ Is the meter suitable if you're pregnant or planning a pregnancy?

✔ Is the meter suitable for the types of other medications that you might be taking? If you require peritoneal dialysis, for example, this need will affect the type of meter you require.

The National Diabetes Services Scheme (NDSS) is funded by the Commonwealth government and offers subsidised test strips to its registered members, so make sure you sign up. If you have private health insurance, your fund may also offer some rebate on a meter if you purchase it, so check with your health fund before you buy.

Talk to your diabetes educator about choosing a blood glucose meter that's right for you. She can cut down the confusion between meters and make the choice simpler. Choose the meter you like, not necessarily the one the doctor likes!

Checking out the alternatives to meters

In Australia, at the time of writing, only one company — Medtronic — offers an alternative device to a meter for measuring your blood glucose levels. This device is known as a *continuous glucose monitoring system* (CGMS).

To get a complete sense of how your blood glucose behaves throughout the day, you could test every minute — or around 1,440 times a day. But who wants to do that? A CGMS uses a sensor that is inserted into the *subcutaneous tissue* (tissue just under the skin) of the abdomen and is then left in place for up to seven days to measure glucose levels over that time (see Figure 9-1). The sensor then transmits the results to a handheld receiver, an insulin pump or saves them so they can be downloaded onto the computer once the sensor has been removed. These monitors can also be programmed to set off an alarm when the blood glucose levels drop too low or go too high, alerting the person wearing the device to take the most appropriate action.

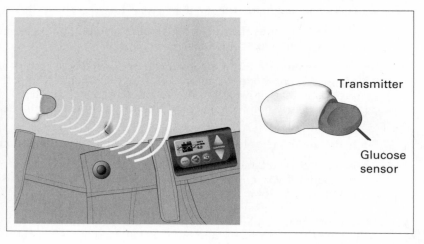

Figure 9-1: A CGMS is inserted into the sub-cutaneous tissue of the abdomen.

Using the CGMS means you're able to see exactly what's happening with your glucose at all hours of the day and night. This can then allow you, your doctor or diabetes educator to better manage your diabetes and, if required, adjust your insulin.

These systems don't replace blood glucose testing meters. The CGMS measures *interstitial fluid* (the fluid found around tissues) rather than blood, so there can be a delay of 5 to 20 minutes between the result that the CGMS is showing you and what your blood glucose levels actually are. This means you still need to test your blood glucose levels before taking any doses of insulin, or if you think you're hypoglycaemic.

While you're wearing the CGMS your diabetes doctor and/or diabetes educator will usually request that you keep a food and activity diary. This involves writing down your blood glucose level, the time you eat, what you're eating and the quantities, along with any activity that you may be doing. Combined with the results from the CGMS, the food and activity diary helps you and your diabetes care team continue to finetune your diabetes management plan.

One of the CGMS offered by Medtronic can be used in conjunction with the company's insulin pump. For the person wearing the Medtronic CGMS and matching insulin pump, some 'talking' between the two is possible. For example, the CGMS sounds an alarm during hypoglycaemia and can switch the pump off during this time if the person with diabetes has not responded. It can then turn the pump back on. (See Chapter 10 for more on insulin pumps.)

CGMS devices are quite expensive. Doctors who specialise in diabetes or staff at diabetes centres may be able to lend a device to patients who they feel may be missing hypoglycaemic events — for example, if the person's blood glucose levels are dropping dangerously low, especially at night, without the person realising it's happened or when there doesn't *appear* to be a pattern in the blood glucose results currently being recorded.

Tracking Your Glucose over Time with Glycosylated Haemoglobin

Individual blood glucose tests are great for deciding how you're doing at one particular moment and what to do to make improvements, but they don't give the big picture — they're just a moment in time. Glucose can change a great deal even in an hour. Even CGMS (see the preceding section) only track levels for up to seven days. What's needed is a test that gives an overall picture of blood glucose levels over many days, weeks or even months. The test that accomplishes this important task is called a glycosylated haemoglobin (HbA1c) test.

Understanding how a HbA1c works

Haemoglobin is a protein that carries oxygen around the body and drops it off wherever it's needed to help in all the chemical reactions that are constantly taking place. The haemoglobin is packaged within red blood cells and it's what gives these cells their colour. Red blood cells live in the bloodstream for between 60 and 90 days.

Glucose attaches in several different ways to the haemoglobin and the total of all the haemoglobin attached to glucose is called *glycohaemoglobin* or *glycosylated haemoglobin*. Once red blood cells become attached to glucose, they stay attached until they die (the cells live for up to three months). As red blood cells die, new ones are produced and glucose can again attach itself to these new cells. The largest proportion of total glycosylated haemoglobin, and therefore the easiest to measure, is known as HbA1c.

The HbA1c test counts the amount of glucose attached to the red blood cells and reports it as a percentage. For example, if 7 out of every 100 red blood cells have glucose attached, the HbA1c result will be 7 per cent. Because glycosylated haemoglobin remains in the blood for up to three months, testing HbA1c levels is a reflection of the glucose control over that whole period.

Blood glucose tests measure the amount of glucose freely circulating in the blood at that given moment, so they use a different unit of measure to the HbA1c test. Blood glucose tests measure millimoles of glucose per litre of blood — or mmol/L. A HbA1c isn't an average of blood glucose levels, but consistently high blood glucose levels will result in more glycosylated red blood cells, thereby increasing HbA1c.

Figure 9-2 shows you the correlation between the HbA1c and blood glucose: A HbA1c of less than 6 per cent corresponds to an average blood glucose of less than 6.6 mmol/L, while a HbA1c of 7 per cent reflects an average blood glucose of 8.3 mmol/L.

Another test similar to HbA1c is *fructosamine*. This test measures blood glucose levels combined with protein in the blood, and reflects the level of blood glucose for the past three weeks. The test can prove to be very useful when you need to know the effect of a treatment change very rapidly — as is the case for pregnant women with gestational diabetes, for example.

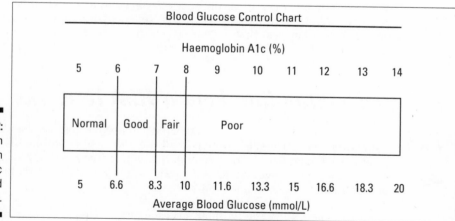

Figure 9-2: Comparison between HbA1c and blood glucose.

Looking at factors that affect HbA1c results

To be accurate, the HbA1c test relies on a three-month lifespan of red blood cells, and this lifespan can sometimes be altered, affecting the HbA1c results.

Circumstances that can affect the lifespan of the red blood cells include the following:

✔ Any illness that affects red blood cell survival

✔ Blood transfusion (including blood donation)

✔ Kidney failure

Unfortunately, not all laboratories conduct the HbA1c test in the same way and this can affect your result. You need to know the normal value in the lab where you had the test. Fortunately, each lab usually has a column on its result form showing the normal values for each test. Still, it makes for a lot of confusion.

Have your HbA1c measured in the same laboratory each time, so that levels can be tracked across the year. This avoids the problem of getting results from different testing methods between laboratories.

Acting on a HbA1c result

Studies have shown that normal HbA1c levels — that is, in people without diabetes — are between 4 and 6 per cent. (Check with the lab where your test is processed for its normal values, and remember that there can be variation within the given normal ranges.)

The Royal Australian College of General Practitioners and Diabetes Australia recommend taking action to control the blood glucose if the HbA1c is 7 per cent or greater. Further monitoring and investigation is required between 6 and 7 per cent; the goal is to achieve less than or equal to 7 per cent.

If you have type 1 diabetes, or type 2 diabetes and are on insulin, your doctor should test you four times a year for HbA1c. A good HbA1c result is highly motivating to keep up good self-care, while a poor result immediately tells you that you need tighter control.

Testing for Ketones in Type 1 Diabetes

When your blood glucose rises above 15.0 mmol/L (or if you are pregnant, have diabetes and your blood glucose is below 3.3 mmol/L), it is a good idea to check for ketones. With a high glucose, it may mean you need more insulin. With a low glucose in pregnancy, it may indicate the need for more carbohydrates in your diet. (Refer to Chapter 6 for more on what ketones are and the symptoms that indicate dangerous levels are building up in your body.)

Finding ketones means that your body has turned to fat as a source of energy. If you find a large amount of ketones, you should contact your GP or diabetes care team as soon as possible for advice.

Two tests can be done for ketones: Blood testing and urine testing.

Testing your blood

Testing the blood is the preferred test for ketones. Ketones appear in the blood first and only appear in the urine after the kidneys have filtered them out of the blood. This means that measuring ketones in the blood tells you the level at the time of the test, and enables you to detect ketones two to four hours earlier than they appear in the urine. Measuring urine levels can also be inaccurate because it can take 8 to 24 hours for the ketones to clear from the urine.

The advantages of blood testing for ketones include the following:

- ✔ You can identify — and treat — dangerous ketone levels a lot quicker.

- ✔ You can determine more accurately whether measures taken to correct high ketone levels are working.

- ✔ If you have type 1 diabetes and are using an insulin pump, you can identify interruptions in insulin flow faster and more accurately than when using blood glucose monitoring.

- ✔ You don't have to pee on a test strip or aim into a small cup, making it much less messy overall!

At the time of writing, only one meter is available in Australia that can test the blood for ketones: The Exceed meter. You can obtain this meter and the required strips from your local National Diabetes Supplies Scheme (NDSS) outlet.

Testing your urine

If you are unable to purchase blood testing strips for ketones, you can use the alternative: Urine testing strips. You take a sample of your urine and then measure ketone levels using a dipstick called a *ketostix*. This is a thin strip of plastic with a pad at the one end that's impregnated with specific chemicals. These chemicals react with ketone bodies and change colour, in a range of rather attractive shades of pinky-purple, depending on the amount of ketones present.

You then check the results by comparing the dipstick to a supplied colour chart — the deeper the colour, the higher the ketone level.

Testing the urine for ketones measures what levels the ketones reached several hours ago, meaning it's not a 'real-time' test. Blood testing is recommended as the preferred option.

Chapter 10

Medications: What You Should Know

. . . .

In This Chapter

▶ Reviewing drugs taken orally

▶ Looking at injecting drugs to help treat type 2 diabetes

▶ Finding out about insulin

▶ Understanding other drugs often prescribed to people with diabetes

▶ Steering clear of dangerous drug combinations

▶ Getting financial assistance with the cost of medication

. . . .

*Y*ou need to take medication if diet and exercise aren't keeping your blood glucose under control. (See Chapters 11 and 12 for tips on using diet and exercise to manage your diabetes.) The good news is that since 1921, when insulin was isolated and used for the first time, and the 1950s, when the first oral medications for type 2 diabetes became available, new classes of drugs have been developed, each lowering blood glucose in its own unique way. (Chapter 20 discusses further developments in drug research).

In this chapter, you become an educated consumer, finding out all you need to know to use medication effectively and safely. Not only can you find out about the medication you're taking and how it works, but also when to take it, how it interacts with other medications and what side effects it may cause. We also advise you on how to use several of these medications together, if necessary, to normalise your blood glucose.

Taking Drugs by Mouth: Oral Agents

Most people with type 2 diabetes start off taking tablets to help control their blood glucose. In this section, we discuss the various oral medications prescribed to help manage diabetes.

Metformin

Metformin is usually the first medication prescribed for most people with type 2 diabetes, and is available in 500-milligram, 850-milligram and 1,000-milligram (1-gram) strengths. Brand names include Diabex, Diaformin, Formet, Glucohexal, Glucomet and Glucophage.

The starting dose for metformin is usually 500 milligrams one to three times daily, and the maximum dose is usually 3 grams per day, taken in two to three doses with meals. However, a new controlled-release preparation of metformin is now available (marketed as Diabex XR or Diaformin XR). These preparations come in 500-milligram and 1,000-milligram tablets and only need to be taken once a day. The maximum dose for the controlled-release preparation is 2 grams per day.

The characteristics of metformin are that it

✔ Lowers blood glucose, mainly by reducing the production of glucose from the liver (hepatic glucose output) and increasing insulin sensitivity; it may slow the uptake of glucose from the intestine

✔ Can cause nausea and diarrhoea; this can be reduced by taking it with food, starting at a low dose and increasing slowly

✔ Might take a couple of weeks to be effective

✔ Does not, by itself (monotherapy), cause hypoglycaemia

✔ When given in combination with a sulphonylurea (see following section), can cause hypoglycaemia; if persistent, the dose of sulphonylurea is reduced.

✔ Is removed from the body by the kidneys; if the kidneys aren't working well, the dose of metformin needs to be reduced

✔ Does not depend on stimulating insulin to work, unlike sulphonylureas

✔ Is often associated with weight loss, possibly from the gastrointestinal irritation or because your stomach can feel more full for longer after a meal

✔ Should not be used when you have significant liver disease, kidney disease or heart failure

✔ Is usually stopped for a day or two before surgery or an x-ray series using a dye

✔ Should not be used by people who drink alcohol excessively

✔ Is not usually recommended for use in women who are pregnant or breastfeeding

Metformin can be a very useful drug, especially when *fasting hyperglycaemia* (high blood glucose upon awakening) is present. Metformin has some positive effects on the blood fats, causing a decrease in triglycerides and LDL cholesterol and an increase in HDL cholesterol.

Metformin occasionally causes a decrease in the absorption of vitamin B12, a vitamin that's important for the blood and the nervous system.

Metformin is also available as a combination drug with other medications to help lower blood glucose. These medications are available in a variety of strengths and can be useful for people stabilised on both drugs by reducing the number of tablets to swallow each day.

Metformin is available in the following combinations:

✔ **Avandamet:** In combination with rosiglitazone

✔ **Glucovance:** In combination with glibenclamide

✔ **Janumet:** In combination with sitagliptin

Sulphonylureas

Scientists discovered sulphonylureas accidentally when it was noticed that soldiers given certain sulphur-containing antibiotics developed symptoms of low blood glucose. Once scientists began to search for the most potent examples of this effect, they came up with several different versions of this drug.

The characteristics of sulphonylureas are that they

✔ Work by making the pancreas release more insulin

✔ Aren't effective in type 1 diabetes (where the pancreas isn't capable of releasing any insulin)

✔ Are all capable of causing hypoglycaemia and weight gain

✔ Should be taken with or immediately before meals

✔ Shouldn't be combined with another medication from this group

✔ Shouldn't be taken by a woman who is pregnant or breastfeeding

✔ Can be fairly potent when given in combination with one of the other classes of oral agents

The original sulphonylureas from the 1950s, the first-generation sulphonylureas, aren't available any more. Some of the more common versions of the second generation available and their brand names are:

✔ **Glibenclamide**, brand names Daonil and Glimel. Glibenclamide comes as a 5-milligram tablet. The usual starting dose is 2.5 milligrams with breakfast, and the maintenance dose is 2.5 to 20 milligrams (twice per day with meals when using a higher dosage). The effect of glibenclamide can last for 18 to 24 hours. Glibenclamide leaves the body equally in the bowel motion and the urine, so patients with either liver or kidney disease are less efficient at eliminating the drug. This means that glibenclamide reaches higher levels in the blood for a longer time, which can cause low blood sugar. This is particularly likely to be a problem in the elderly. Glibenclamide is used much less often than the other sulphonylureas because it's more likely than the other drugs in this group to cause hypoglycaemia.

✔ **Gliclazide**, brand names Diamicron and Glyade. Gliclazide comes in 80-milligram tablets and its effect lasts for 12 to 16 hours. The starting dose is 40 milligrams and can be given once or twice daily up to 320 milligrams per day (with a maximum single dose of 160 milligrams). Both brands now offer a modified-release version of the same drug, marketed as Diamicron MR or Glyade MR. These versions last for 16 to 24 hours, so they only need to be taken once a day. The modified-release formulations come in 60-milligram tablets and are given in a single daily dose, starting at 30 milligrams and with the maximum dosage being 120 milligrams. These tablets may be broken in half but must not be crushed or chewed.

✔ **Glimepiride**, brand name Amaryl. Glimepiride comes in 1-, 2- and 4-milligram tablets. The effect of glimepiride lasts for 24 hours so it's given once a day. The usual starting dose is 1 milligram with breakfast. If control of blood glucose is not adequate after one to two weeks, the dose can be increased by 1 milligram at one- to two-week intervals until a satisfactory maintenance dose is reached.

✔ **Glipizide**, brand names Melizide and Minidiab. Glipizide comes as a 5-milligram tablet. The starting dose is 2.5 milligrams, and up to 40 milligrams can be given daily in several doses (doses should be at least twice daily when using more than 15 milligrams per day). The effect of glipizide lasts for six to eight hours, so it's often preferred for the elderly.

Acarbose

Acarbose, brand name Glucobay, blocks the action of an enzyme in the gut called *alpha glucosidase*. This enzyme is responsible for breaking down complex carbohydrates into smaller molecules like glucose and fructose so that they can be absorbed. The result is that the rate in the rise of glucose in the bloodstream is slowed after meals. These carbohydrates are eventually broken down by bacteria lower down in the intestine and produce a lot of flatulence, abdominal pain and diarrhoea, which are the major drawbacks of this drug.

The main characteristics of acarbose are

- ✔ Availability in 50-milligram and 100-milligram strengths.

- ✔ The tablets can be swallowed whole at the beginning of a meal or chewed with the first few mouthfuls of food.

- ✔ The recommended starting dose is 50 milligrams once daily with a gradual increase to 50 milligrams three times daily. This dose can be increased to 100 milligrams three times daily after six to eight weeks, depending on the response; the maximum daily dose is 600 milligrams.

- ✔ It doesn't cause hypoglycaemia when used alone but can in combination with sulphonylureas. If hypoglycaemia is persistent, the dose of sulphonylurea is decreased.

- ✔ It doesn't require insulin for its activity.

- ✔ Many people don't like it because of the gastrointestinal side effects.

- ✔ The lowering of glucose and HbA1c (refer to Chapter 9) is modest at most.

Many doctors have not found much use for acarbose. We have tried it on a number of patients, and even though they started at a low dose and gradually built up to a more effective level, they complained about flatulence and abdominal pain and asked us to take them off the drug. Because we weren't seeing much change in the blood glucose, we didn't object.

Some people have found that using acarbose enhances the effects of glibenclamide (refer to the previous section on sulphonylureas). Acarbose has also been successful when used in the prevention of diabetes in impaired glucose tolerance; however, it is not available for that purpose in Australia.

Because acarbose acts by blocking the breakdown of complex carbohydrates, hypoglycaemia occurring with acarbose and sulphonylurea combinations must be treated with a preparation of glucose such as Glucojel jellybeans.

Thiazolidinediones (the glitazones)

The glitazones are the first group of drugs for type 2 diabetes that directly target insulin resistance by causing changes within the muscle and fat cells where the insulin resistance occurs. This means that the body doesn't have to make as much insulin to control the blood glucose. These changes take several weeks to occur and some people may not respond at all. Because they improve insulin resistance, the greatest effect on blood glucose is shown after eating.

Two glitazones are available in Australia: Pioglitazone and rosiglitazone.

Pioglitazone

Pioglitazone (brand name Actos) has the following features:

✔ It is available in 15-, 30- and 45-milligram tablets.

✔ The starting dose is 15 to 30 milligrams once daily; the dose can be increased after six to eight weeks if necessary to a maximum of 45 milligrams daily.

✔ It may also help your blood fats.

Rosiglitazone

Rosiglitazone (brand name Avandia) has the following features:

✔ It is available in 2-, 4- and 8-milligram tablets.

✔ It may be given once or twice per day, with or without food.

✔ The recommended starting dose is 4 milligrams per day; this dose can be increased to 8 milligrams per day after six to eight weeks if greater control of blood glucose is required.

✔ It is also available as a combination tablet with metformin (marketed as Avandamet) in a number of different combinations of strengths.

Possible side effects from using thiazolidinediones

The glitazone drugs can, however, have associated problems. They

✔ Can cause fluid retention and swelling of the ankles in some people, especially the elderly. This can cause problems in people who are at risk of congestive heart disease, so heart function may need to be monitored. Tell your doctor if you notice any swelling, breathlessness or weight gain.

✔ May cause hypoglycaemia if combined with other medication for diabetes. (They are unlikely to cause hypoglycaemia if used on their own.)

✔ May increase the chance of broken bones in the upper arm, hand or foot; while this may be more of a problem if you have osteoporosis, it's always important to do what you can to keep your bones strong.

✔ Can worsen macular oedema; make sure you have your regular eye checks and tell your doctor if you notice changes in your vision.

In addition to the possible side effects included in the preceding list, rosiglitazone has been associated with further risks:

✔ Some studies have raised the possibility of an increased risk of death from heart attack in people taking rosiglitazone; for this reason its use is now carefully monitored.

✔ Rosiglitazone isn't approved for use with insulin. If pioglitazone is used with insulin, it will need to be monitored closely due to the chance of fluid retention and heart failure

Studies have shown that no dosage adjustments are required in patients with kidney impairment.

A related thiazolidinedione drug, troglitazone, was taken off the market because it caused liver damage in some people. Rosiglitazone and pioglitazone seem to be free of these liver problems. However, before starting treatment, you should have a liver function test to measure your liver enzymes, and then have these tested periodically.

Glitazone drugs should not be taken by women who are pregnant or breastfeeding.

Unexpected side effects, such as unintended pregnancies, have occurred in women of child-bearing age who take glitazones. As a consequence of insulin resistance, many such women have reduced fertility; when they take glitazones, their fertility may improve and they may become pregnant.

Generally, glitazones are used in conjunction with other oral hypoglycaemic agents. This type of regimen is initiated in people with type 2 diabetes in whom diet and exercise and other tablets are not successful and the blood glucose is still mildly to moderately elevated.

Glitazones are only available on the Pharmaceutical Benefits Scheme through an authority script. Strict criteria for use have been laid down by the Australian government.

Repaglinide

Repaglinide, brand name Novonorm, belongs to the group of drugs called *meglitinides*, which are chemically unrelated to the sulphonylureas but work by squeezing more insulin out of the pancreas, just like the sulphonylureas do. Repaglinide, however, is taken just before meals to stimulate insulin for only that meal.

The characteristics of repaglinide are that it

- Is available as 0.5, 1 and 2 milligram tablets taken just before or up to 30 minutes before meals; if you're skipping a meal, don't take the tablet

- Has a starting dose of 0.5 milligrams with a mild elevation of blood glucose or 1 or 2 milligrams if the initial blood glucose is higher; the dose may be doubled once a week to a maximum of 4 milligrams before meals (daily maximum of 12 milligrams)

- Can cause hypoglycaemia, because it acts through insulin

- Is not recommended for use in women who are pregnant or breastfeeding

- Should not be used with the sulphonylureas but can be combined with metformin; use in combination with rosiglitazone or pioglitazone has not been studied

- Lowers the blood glucose and the HbA1c effectively when used in combination with metformin

- Is mostly broken down in the liver and leaves the body in the bowel movement; if liver disease is present, the dose has to be adjusted downward

- Must be monitored closely when used by people with kidney impairment, despite the lack of excretion through the kidneys, with increases in the dose made more carefully

Because this drug is only available on a private script, it is expensive.

Dipeptidyl peptidase-IV inhibitors

The dipeptidyl peptidase-IV (DPP-IV) inhibitors belong to the newest group of drugs available for type 2 diabetes called *incretin enhancers*. When you eat food, hormones called incretins are secreted from the gut. Incretins stimulate the pancreas to produce insulin and reduce the amount of glucose made by the liver. The DPP-IV inhibitors slow the breakdown of incretins so they can work more effectively.

DPP-IV inhibitors have only recently been released in Australia, so keep an eye out for more new drugs from this group as they hit the diabetes market.

At the time of writing, two members of this group are available in Australia on the Pharmaceutical Benefits Scheme with an authority prescription: Sitagliptin and vildagliptin.

Sitagliptin

The characteristics of sitagliptin (brand name Januvia) are that it

- ✓ Comes in 25, 50 and 100 milligram tablets
- ✓ Is usually taken as a 100-milligram dose once daily, with or without food
- ✓ Is mainly excreted in the urine; doses are reduced if kidney function is impaired
- ✓ Comes also as a combination tablet with metformin (marketed as Janumet), which is taken twice daily with or after food

Vildagliptin

The characteristics of vildagliptin (brand name Galvus) are that it

- ✓ Comes in 50 milligram tablets
- ✓ Can be taken once or twice daily with or without food
- ✓ Should not be used by people with renal impairment

Possible side effects from using DPP-IV inhibitors

Because DPP-IV inhibitors are a new class of medication, the long-term safety is unknown. Some known adverse effects include the following:

- ✓ Allergic reactions such as a rash or swelling have been reported rarely; see you doctor if you notice any such symptoms
- ✓ Headache
- ✓ Infections of the *nasopharyngeal* area (the area of the throat behind the nose) and upper respiratory tract infections, which produce symptoms similar to a cold
- ✓ Pancreatitis has been reported but it's unclear if it was caused by these medications

Because the DPP-IV inhibitors only work in response to food, they're unlikely to cause hypoglycaemia when used with metformin; however, the chance of hypoglycaemia is greater if combined with a sulphonylurea. They have a neutral effect on weight.

Oral agents combined

As you might expect, taking one oral agent alone often doesn't control the blood glucose to the point where the chance of complications of diabetes is reduced.

No drug should be taken as a convenient way of avoiding the basic diet and exercise that are the keys to good control (see Chapters 11 and 12 for information about these crucial factors).

Everyone is different, so it's up to you and your doctor to decide on the most appropriate oral agents for you.

The Royal Australian College of General Practitioners and Diabetes Australia recommend starting with metformin for most people with type 2 diabetes. If blood glucose isn't adequately controlled, a second tablet is usually added; which drug is chosen depends on your individual circumstances.

Current medical belief is that the pancreas gradually fails to make insulin in type 2 diabetes and that most patients need insulin sooner or later (see the sidebar 'Combining insulin and oral agents in type 2 diabetes').

Getting Under Your Skin: Injecting Incretin Mimetics

A new group of drugs available for people with type 2 diabetes is the *incretin mimetics*. When you eat food, incretin hormones stimulate the pancreas to produce insulin and reduce the production of glucagon, resulting in an increase in glucose uptake by muscle and a reduction in the amount of glucose made by the liver. Artificial incretin mimetics work by copying this process.

Exenatide (marketed in Australia as Byetta) is one of these agents. The drug results in increased insulin production in response to food, a reduction in glucose made by the liver, and a slowing of glucose absorption by slowing stomach emptying and reducing appetite. Unlike the DPP inhibitors (refer to the section 'Dipeptidyl peptidase-IV inhibitors' earlier in this section), exenatide is only available as a subcutaneous (beneath the skin) injection.

Exenatide has the following characteristics:

✔ It's available as a prefilled, disposable pen injection device in 5 or 10 milligram per dose strengths.

✔ It's stored in the fridge and each pen contains enough to last for a month.

✔ The dose is 5 to 10 milligram injected under the skin one hour *before* breakfast and dinner; it should not be used after a meal.

✔ Because it slows stomach emptying, it can affect the absorption of other medicines; take other medicines one hour before taking exenatide to reduce this effect.

✔ It's associated with a small weight loss.

Hypoglycaemia is unlikely unless exenatide is used in combination with a sulphonylurea.

Because exenatide is a new medication, the long-term safety is unknown at the time of writing. Short-term effects such as nausea, vomiting and diarrhoea are known to be common, but for many people these symptoms settle down in a week or two. Starting with a small dose and increasing after a few weeks also helps reduce these short-term effects. Pancreatitis and kidney problems have been rarely reported but it's as yet unknown if they were caused by exenatide.

Unfortunately, some people need to stop taking exenatide because the nausea caused by the drug doesn't disappear and this side effect is too unpleasant for them to tolerate. If this happens to you, see your doctor to discuss alternatives — don't just stop taking the drug!

Introducing Insulin

If you're a person with type 1 diabetes, insulin is your saviour. If you have type 2 diabetes, you may need insulin late in the course of your disease. Insulin is a great drug, but it must be injected under the skin at the present time.

Until a few years ago, insulin could only be obtained by extracting it from the pancreas of cows, pigs, salmon and some other animals. This wasn't entirely satisfactory because those insulins are slightly different from human insulin. Using them resulted in an immune reaction in the blood and certain skin reactions. The preparation was purified but there were always tiny amounts of impurities. In 1978, researchers were able to trick bacteria called *E. coli* into making human insulin. All insulin is now pure human insulin.

Reviewing the types of insulin

In the human body, insulin is constantly responding to ups and downs in the blood glucose. No simple device is currently available to measure the blood glucose and deliver insulin as the pancreas does. In order to copy the body's production of insulin as closely as possible, different forms of insulin were developed to work in different time frames. These forms of insulin include

✔ **Rapid onset, ultra short-acting insulin (Humalog (lispro) manufactured by Eli Lilly, NovoRapid (aspart) from Novo Nordisk and Apidra (glulisine) from Sanofi Aventis):** The rapid-acting insulins begin to lower the glucose within five minutes after administration, peak at about one hour, and are no longer active after four to five hours. This is a great advance because it frees people with diabetes to allow them to inject just when they eat. With the previous short-acting insulin (neutral insulin), a person had to inject and wait to eat for 30 minutes (hardly convenient!). Because their activity begins and ends so quickly, rapid-acting insulins don't cause hypoglycaemia as often as the earlier preparations.

✔ **Short-acting neutral or soluble insulin (Actrapid from Novo Nordisk, Humulin R from Eli Lilly and Hypurin Neutral from Aventis):** Neutral insulin takes 30 minutes to start to lower the glucose, peaks at three hours and is gone within six to eight hours. This insulin is the preparation that was used before meals to keep the glucose low until the next meal. These insulins are rapidly fading in popularity because the ultra short-acting insulins suit most people better.

✔ **Intermediate-acting Isophane/NPH insulin (Humulin NPH from Eli Lilly and Protaphane from Novo Nordisk):** This form of insulin begins to lower the glucose within two hours of administration and continues its activity for 16 to 24 hours. The purpose of this kind of insulin is to provide a level of active insulin constantly in the body. However, it does contain a distinctive peak in its action, making it less popular for some people now that we have some peakless long-acting insulins.

✔ **Long-acting insulins (glargine (Lantus) from Sanofi-Aventis and insulin detemir (Levemir) from Novo Nordisk):** Glargine insulin has an onset between one and two hours after injection. Its activity lasts for 24 hours without a specific peak activity. This assists in controlling the blood glucose levels over the entire day. Because of its smooth and more predictable activity, glargine is less likely to cause low blood glucose levels at night. Insulin detemir has an onset of three to four hours and a duration of 12 to 24 hours. It may be used twice a day in some people with type 1 diabetes to ensure a full, 24-hour coverage. The Australian PBS does not allow insulin detemir to be prescribed for people with type 2 diabetes who require insulin.

✔ **Premixed insulins:** These contain combinations of different short- and long-acting insulins in different percentages. These insulins can be helpful for people who have trouble giving multiple daily injections, have poor eyesight or are stable on a preparation that doesn't change. The usual percentage combinations are:

- Neutral 30 per cent and isophane 70 per cent (Humulin 30/70 and Mixtard 30/70)

- Neutral 50 per cent and isophane 50 per cent (Mixtard 50/50)

- Lispro 25 per cent and lispro protamine 75 per cent (Humalog Mix25)

- Lispro 50 per cent and lispro protamine 50 per cent (Humalog Mix50)

- Aspart 30 per cent and aspart protamine 70 per cent (NovoMix30)

Understanding common features of all insulins

A few things are common to all insulins:

✔ Insulin may be kept at room temperature for four weeks or in the refrigerator until the expiration date printed on the label. After four weeks at room temperature, it should be discarded.

✔ Insulin doesn't take too well to excessive heat, such as direct sunlight, or to excessive cold. Protect your insulin against these conditions or it will lose its action.

✔ You can safely give an insulin injection through clothing.

✔ Various needle sizes are available. Talk to your diabetes nurse educator to discuss what type of needle is best for you.

✔ Used syringes and needles should be disposed of in an Australian Safety Standards approved sharps container, which is puncture-proof and sealed shut before disposal. These containers can be obtained from the Australian Diabetes Council (in NSW), Diabetes Australia offices in other states, and some local councils, depending on which state or territory you live in.

Where you inject the insulin helps to determine how predictably it will work. For example, insulin injected into the abdomen is absorbed more regularly and in a more predictable way. If you inject into the arms and legs or the buttocks, this predictability is lost and other factors (such as how much the area is being exercised) come into play, making blood glucose levels more erratic. Also, if you use the same site repeatedly, the absorption rate may change as you may develop fatty, hard lumps at the injection site.

The accuracy of your insulin dose is dependent on the accuracy of your injection technique. Make sure you rotate the location of your injection site and learn how to give the injection from an expert — a credentialled diabetes nurse educator!

For many people with diabetes, the timing of insulin injections is also important to help make blood glucose control more predictable. Check with your diabetes care team for advice on which of your insulins need to be taken at the same time and which ones you can be more flexible with (if any!).

Conducting intensive insulin treatment

Intensive insulin treatment is essential in type 1 diabetes if you hope to prevent the complications of the disease. This means measuring your blood glucose at least before each meal and at bedtime, and using both rapid-acting and intermediate-acting insulin to keep the blood glucose between 4.4 and 5.5 mmol/L before meals and less than 8 mmol/L after eating. How you do this is the subject of this section.

In the human body (except in type 1 diabetes), a small amount of circulating insulin is always in the bloodstream and, after eating, insulin increases temporarily to control the glucose in the meal. Intensive insulin treatment attempts to mirror the normal human pancreas as much as possible.

In intensive insulin treatment, a long-acting insulin provides a constant level of circulating insulin and rapid-acting insulin covers each meal. The dose of rapid-acting insulin is determined by the expected grams of carbohydrates in the meal about to be taken plus the blood glucose at that moment. Your doctor or diabetes educator will work with you to determine how much insulin to take for a given situation. Each person is different, and this must be individualised.

When you use the carbohydrates in the meal to determine the insulin dose, it is called *carbohydrate counting*. You can quickly work out how much carbohydrate is in each meal if you know how large or small your serving size is and how much carbohydrate is in it. Your specialist diabetes dietitian can go over your food preferences and show you how many carbohydrates are in them. The dietitian can also show you where to find carbohydrate quantities for any foods that you might eat. (See Chapter 11 for more on counting carbohydrates when you have type 1 diabetes. See Chapter 12 for more on working exercise in with your insulin.)

Combining insulin and oral agents in type 2 diabetes

Sometimes the characteristics of the currently available oral agents don't provide the tight control needed to avoid complications. This is particularly true after many years of type 2 diabetes. Then insulin may be required. Insulin may be added in a number of ways, but often an injection of long-acting insulin at bedtime is all that is needed to start the day under control and continue it with oral agents. Tablets may control the daytime glucose very well after eating, but the first morning glucose may need the overnight injection of insulin.

As type 2 diabetes progresses, the oral agents may be less effective, and insulin is taken more often. Two injections a day of a premixed insulin may do the trick. Usually you take two-thirds of the dose in the morning and one-third before dinner — because you need rapid-acting insulin to control the dinner carbohydrates. This combination is especially valuable in elderly people with diabetes, where the tightest level of control is not being sought because the expected lifespan of the person is shorter than the time necessary to develop complications. In this person, doctors want to prevent problems like frequent urination leading to loss of sleep, or vaginal infections, so they give enough insulin to treat this but not so much that this frail, elderly patient is having hypoglycaemia on a frequent basis. Alternatively, a rapid-acting insulin may be added at mealtimes.

When a second injection of insulin is needed, tablets from the sulphonylureas or repaglinide group of drugs are usually stopped. Because the pancreas is no longer able to make enough insulin, these drugs are unable to work well enough. At this point, metformin is continued to keep working on the person's insulin sensitivity and so minimise the dose of insulin needed.

Adjusting insulin when travelling

With the increasing use of the new long-acting, peakless insulins glargine and insulin detemir, the problems of adjusting insulin with air travel are a thing of the past. However, it's a little trickier if you are using the premixed insulins.

Because each person has a different insulin requirement and long-distance travel arrangements differ, see your endocrinologist or diabetes educator several weeks before travelling to discuss what you should do about your doses when flying.

Many of the insulin companies provide specialised insulated carry bags to keep your insulin cold while travelling, and you can pick some up from your local diabetes centre. Always take more insulin than you think you'll need. If travelling with a companion, split your insulin between you in case your hand luggage gets lost or stolen.

Insulin should not be packed in your check-in luggage as the temperature in the hold is too cold and the insulin may freeze. Frozen (and then defrosted) insulin is unusable.

When travelling overseas, all people with diabetes — on insulin or not — will need a letter from their doctor listing the medications they are on and the current doses. This information can be requested by customs officials to crosscheck with the medications packed in your luggage. A letter outlining that you have diabetes and will be carrying blood glucose testing equipment, needle tips and hypoglycaemia treatment is also a good idea to prevent possible misunderstandings when you're found to have 'pointy things' or volumes greater than 100 millilitres in your hand luggage!

Delivering insulin with a syringe or a pen

Devices for delivering insulin have undergone many changes from when they were first used by people with diabetes. Syringes are very rarely used and have been replaced by insulin pens. The exception to this may be in some hospitals and aged care facilities.

The needle tips have also been subject to vast improvements over the years. The current needles are extremely fine and come in several lengths. Your diabetes educator can provide you with the most appropriate needles for your individual needs. Needles are supplied free of charge in most Australian states and territories for people with a National Diabetes Services Scheme (NDSS) card.

Two types of pens are available in Australia:

 ✔ **Pens that you load with a cartridge of insulin.** Types available include NovoPen 3 and 4 for Novo Nordisk insulin cartridges; Humapen, Luxura and Memoir for Lilly insulin cartridges; and ClickSTAR for Sanofi Aventis insulin cartridges.

 ✔ **Disposable pens that are preloaded for you and discarded when the insulin is finished.** Options available in Australia include FlexPen, Innolet or NovoLet for NovoNordisk insulins; KwikPen for Lilly insulins; and SoloSTAR for Sanofi Aventis insulins.

Not all pen devices come in all types of insulin; you need to work with your GP and diabetes educator to determine which is best for you.

The number of units you have dialled up for use is displayed in a window on the pen. Each unit (or sometimes each set of two units) is accompanied by a clicking sound so that, if you are visually impaired, you can hear the number of units that you've dialled up for delivery. If you dial up too many units, the pen allows you to reset the dial and start again without wasting insulin. All pens contain 300 units of insulin.

Depending on the pen, you can deliver up to 80 units of insulin in one go and you screw on a new needle as needed.

Delivering insulin with an external pump

Insulin pumps or continuous subcutaneous insulin infusions (CSII) are increasingly being used in Australia by people with type 1 diabetes, both children and adults.

These devices are small, battery-powered, computerised pumps that are about the size of a pager (see Figure 10-1). You can wear an insulin pump clipped onto your belt, in your pocket or bra, or in a pouch. The pump holds a syringe (or reservoir) filled with rapid-acting insulin and is programmed to give small amounts of insulin through an *infusion set* (a thin piece of plastic tubing attached to the pump at one end and with a small needle at the other end).

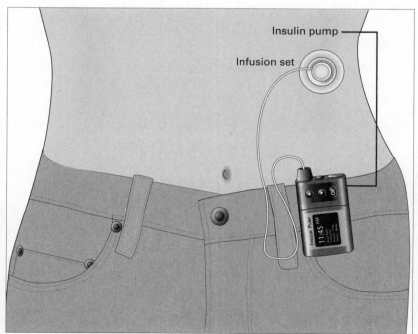

Insulin pump

Infusion set

Figure 10-1:
An insulin pump is small and can be clipped onto your belt.

You attach an insulin pump by inserting the needle at the end of the infusion set into the fatty tissue just under your skin. You then remove the needle, leaving the *cannula* (a small flexible silicon tube) under the skin. The cannula is made of silicon because this has only a small chance of causing allergic reactions, and becomes very flexible and comfortable when at body temperature.

Pump therapy is not for everyone. Pumps are expensive and you need to work closely with your diabetes care team to learn how to use the pump and commit to follow-up care and education. For more information about insulin pumps, and working out whether using one is right for you, see Appendix A.

Finding aids to insulin delivery

Those of you still using the old needle and syringe method will want to know about the numerous aids that can make it easier for you to take your insulin:

- **Automatic injectors (B-D Inject-Ease Automatic Injector and NovoPen 3 PenMate):** These devices are spring-loaded. They enable you to put your syringe, NovoPen 3 or NovoPen 3 Demi in the holder, place it against your skin and press a button that puts the needle through the skin quickly — and you've administered the insulin. The needle is hidden from view when injecting, making automatic injectors useful devices for those who dislike seeing the needle.

- **Syringe magnifiers (B-D Magni-Guide):** These clip onto the neck of the insulin vial and magnify the syringe barrel and scale, which helps visually impaired people to administer insulin.

Contact your local diabetes educator to find out more about these devices.

Other Common Medications

Minimising the chance of long-term complications of diabetes involves more than just looking after your blood glucose! Good control of blood pressure and blood lipids (cholesterol and other fats) are important and your doctor may suggest medication to help achieve this. Medication may also be prescribed to help reduce the chance of a heart attack or stroke, or to help with weight loss.

Remembering to take all your medications as intended can be difficult, especially when they don't immediately make you feel any different. To help you keep track, make a list of all your medicines (names and strengths), when to take them and what they are for. Your pharmacist can help you prepare this and help with working out a routine that fits with your lifestyle — and answer any questions you may have.

Antihypertensives (medicines for lowering blood pressure)

People with diabetes are more likely to have high blood pressure than people without diabetes. Often, diet and lifestyle efforts aren't enough to get blood pressure to the treatment targets (refer to Chapter 7 for more on treatment targets for blood pressure), so medications may be prescribed. Because these medications act slightly differently, they can be combined to work together, meaning you may end up taking three or more medicines from different groups to help you achieve a target blood pressure.

Many antihypertensives are available in combination tablets, which helps reduce the number of tablets you need each day. Talk with your GP to see if a suitable combination is available for you.

Some common blood pressure medicines are

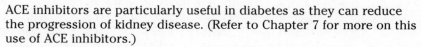

- ✔ **ACE inhibitors.** These medicines reduce the amount of a chemical called *angiotensin* in the body, allowing the blood vessels to relax and widen to reduce blood pressure. They may raise potassium levels, and/or cause a dry cough and an allergic reaction; talk with your doctor if you notice swelling, a rash or any other symptom that you think may be related to your medication.

  ACE inhibitors are particularly useful in diabetes as they can reduce the progression of kidney disease. (Refer to Chapter 7 for more on this use of ACE inhibitors.)

- ✔ **Angiotensin receptor blockers.** Like ACE inhibitors, this group also reduces the amount of angiotensin in the body, but at a different point. Angiotensin receptor blockers have similar side effects to ACE inhibitors, although the allergies are less likely to occur. They also reduce the progression of kidney disease in diabetes.

- ✔ **Beta blockers.** These medicines work by blocking beta one receptors in the heart, reducing the work done by the heart and stopping the blood vessels from tightening. Beta blockers can cause breathlessness in people with asthma and mask some signs of hypoglycaemia.

✔ **Calcium channel blockers.** These medicines block the use of calcium in the blood vessels, allowing them to relax. They have been shown to cause ankle swelling; if you notice this symptom, ask your doctor about taking a different blood pressure medication.

✔ **Thiazide and related diuretics (fluid tablets).** When used in low doses for blood pressure these medications work mainly by relaxing blood vessels. They can cause too many salts, such as potassium, to be lost in the urine; talk to your doctor about monitoring these levels if you are on this medication.

All antihypertensive medications can cause low blood pressure, so be careful particularly when getting up from lying down or sitting.

Drugs for dyslipidemia (abnormal levels of fats in the blood)

In addition to switching to a low-fat diet and increasing exercise, medication may also be required to manage the levels of fats in your blood; several different groups of medicines are now available to do this. Again, you may need to be on more than one type of medication to help you reach your desired targets.

Drugs commonly available to help with lowering the levels of fats in your blood include the following:

✔ **Ezetimibe.** This medication works by blocking the absorption of cholesterol in the gut. It is taken once a day and may be added if a statin alone is not effective enough. Like the statins, ezetimibe may also cause muscle pain and weakness; it can also cause diarrhoea.

✔ **Fibrates.** This group of medication works mainly by reducing triglyceride levels (one of the damaging fats; refer to Chapter 7 for more on the different types of fats). Fibrates can also cause muscle pain or weakness and liver reactions (this may be more likely if you're also taking a statin), increase the sensitivity of your skin to sun exposure, and may also cause stomach upsets.

✔ **Fish Oils.** Fish oils contain two active ingredients: Eicosapentaenoic acid (EPA) and docosahexaenoic acid (DHA), which can lower triglyceride levels in the blood. To be effective, you need to take 1.2 to 5 grams of these active ingredients each day. Fish oil supplements that you buy vary widely in their levels of EPA and DHA, so read the label carefully to determine how many capsules you need to meet your recommended daily target.

✔ **Statins.** This group is also known as *HMG-CoA reductase inhibitors* because they block the HMG-CoA reductase enzyme, needed for making cholesterol in the body. They're the most common medication prescribed to improve lipid levels, and are usually taken once a day. These medications can cause a rise in liver enzymes, which your GP can monitor, and may cause muscle pain or weakness; see your GP if you experience these symptoms.

Antiplatelet medication

These medicines are used to reduce the likelihood of clots forming in your blood vessels, which could result in a heart attack or a stroke.

Antiplatelet medications include the following:

✔ **Aspirin.** Used in doses of 100 milligram or 150 milligram once per day, this medication can be bought over the counter without a prescription. Aspirin may cause stomach upsets and increase the likelihood of bleeding.

✔ **Clopidogrel.** This medication may be used if you can't tolerate aspirin or if you have another heart condition. A 75-milligram tablet is taken once daily.

Weight loss medication

People with type 2 diabetes are often overweight or obese, and so, in conjunction with a low-kilojoule diet high in fruit and vegetables and increased exercise, may also be prescribed medications to help with weight loss.

The only scientifically proven weight loss medications available in Australia at the time of writing that we would recommend are:

✔ **Orlistat (marketed as Xenical).** This medication works by blocking the absorption of dietary fat in the gut. You take a 120-milligram capsule at the same time as or up to one hour after your three main meals. You should not take the dose if you're skipping a meal or if the meal doesn't contain fat.

Orlistat can be purchased over the counter but is expensive; check with your GP or diabetes care team to see if you qualify for an authority prescription.

✔ **Phentermine (marketing as Duromine or Metermine).** This drug is a sympathetic nervous system stimulant with some appetite suppressant activity. It is taken once daily at breakfast for a maximum of 12 weeks. It has a limited use as it may cause overstimulation, resulting in high blood pressure, heart problems, insomnia, agitation, rash and impotence. It increases the effect of alcohol and may affect your ability to drive.

While Duromine has been available in Australia for many years, it's not commonly prescribed because of its rather unpleasant side effects. The drug is also addictive, so can only be used for three months. It is best used under strict supervision and only if you don't have high blood pressure or heart problems.

Weight loss drugs only work while you take them. As soon as you stop taking them, your body returns to normal and, unless you can continue a low-kilojoule diet without the help of the drugs, you'll often put any weight lost straight back on.

See Chapter 11 for more discussion on diet and the use and effectiveness of weight loss medications.

'Miracle' preparations for weight loss are commonly available without a prescription but often lack good evidence to show that they work and may have side effects. See Chapter 21 for a further discussion of these preparations.

Avoiding Drug Interactions

A person with diabetes may be taking several different drugs, which may interact and cause drug toxicity problems. Sometimes (believe it or not) even your GP isn't aware of the interactions of common drugs. You need to know the names of all the drugs you take (both the brand names and the names of the medicine it contains) and whether they affect one another.

Many common medications also raise the blood glucose, sometimes bringing out a diabetic tendency that might otherwise not have been recognised.

Drugs that may raise blood glucose include the following:

✔ Chlorpromazine (Largactil), clozapine (Clozaril), haloperidol (Serenace), olanzapine (Zyprexa), paliperidone (Invega), quetiapine (Seroquel), respiridone (Risperdal), amitriptyline (Tryptanol), clomipramine (Anafranil), dothiepin (Prothiaden), doxepin (Sinequan, Deptran), imipramine (Tofranil), nortriptyline (Allegron) and trimipramine (Surmontil), used for mental health conditions

- Colaspase or L-asparaginase (Leunase), fludarabine (Fludara) and Nilotinib (Tasigna), used to treat some types of cancer

- Corticosteroids, such as prednisone, used to block autoimmune conditions

- Cyclosporin, everolimus, sirolimus and tacrolimus, used to prevent organ rejection, and temsirolimus, used to treat some types of cancer

- Interferon alfa (Roferon-A), used to treat hepatitis and some forms of cancer

- Isoniazid, used as a treatment for tuberculosis

- Isotetnoin, used for severe acne

- Nicotinic acid in high doses, used to lower cholesterol

- Phenytoin (Dilantin), used to prevent seizures

- Protease inhibitors including atazanavir (Reyataz), darunavir (Prezista), fosamprenavir (Telzir), indinavir (Crixivan), lopinavir with ritonavir (Kaletra), ritonavir (Norvir), sasquinavir (Invirase) and tipranivir (Aptivus), used as antiretroviral medication for HIV infection

- Rifampicin, used as an antibiotic, can increase the metabolism of glibenclamide, gliclazide, repaglinide and thiazolidinediones, making them less effective at lowering blood sugar

Some common drugs or medications also lower the blood glucose. The most important of these include the following:

- Alcohol can lower the blood glucose, particularly when taken without food.

- Aspirin, in high doses

- Gemfibrozil, used to treat disorders of fat, and the antibiotic trimethoprim increase the effect of repaglinide and thiazolidinedines, which may cause a lowering of blood glucose.

If you're taking these drugs, the change in your blood glucose may not be significant. The best idea is to monitor your blood glucose if you start a new medication and discuss any changes with your GP.

Getting Help with the Costs of Diabetes

Diabetes can be expensive, especially if you need several drugs to control your blood glucose. Many diabetes medications have been listed on the government-funded Pharmaceutical Benefits Scheme, which provides drugs at subsidised prices. Most diabetes medications (including insulin and some oral hypoglycaemic agents) are listed on the scheme. Others such as repaglinide are not, which makes them very expensive options.

Some medications may be available in cheaper brands, often called *generics*. They contain the same medication and have to meet the same Australian standards, so are safe to take for most people.

Don't be confused by different brand names for what is really the same drug. All medicines are labelled with the name of the drug they contain, so just make sure you know what this drug is.

Diabetes Australia operates the Commonwealth Government's National Diabetes Services Scheme (NDSS), which subsidises the cost of test strips and provides free needles and syringes. You can register at the Australian Diabetes Council (in NSW) or Diabetes Australia in other states. A special form must be signed by your doctor or credentialed diabetes educator to receive a free benefits card. All people with diabetes who have a Medicare card are entitled to be registered with the NDSS scheme and receive the associated discounts.

Members of the Australian Diabetes Council (in NSW) and Diabetes Australia (in other states) also receive discounts on such items as glucose tablets, foot moisturisers, swabs, glucose meters and control solutions, insulin-injecting devices, sweeteners, recipe books and informative books and videos. Membership for these groups can be arranged by phoning the relevant group in your state (see Chapter 24 for website details, where contact numbers can be found).

Your health insurance company may also provide rebates on meters, depending on your level of cover.

Chapter 11

Healthy Eating in Diabetes

· ·

In This Chapter

▶ Focusing on the dietary needs of people with type 2 diabetes

▶ Taking action to check and reduce your weight when you have type 2 diabetes

▶ Reviewing the special needs of people with type 1 diabetes

▶ Understanding the effect of vitamins, minerals, water and alcohol on all people with diabetes

· ·

*T*he nutritional needs of human beings are the same regardless of whether or not you have diabetes. However, when making adjustments to your diet to accommodate your diabetes, differences exist between the advice for those with type 1 and that for those with type 2 diabetes.

In this chapter, you find out much that you need to know to make your diet work for you, not only to improve your diabetes and control your blood glucose, but also to generally feel that you have an improved quality of life. Every person is unique, however, so make sure you also see a specialist diabetes dietitian, who can give you individualised advice. Please note that we've divided this chapter based on whether you have type 1 or type 2 diabetes. Where similarities occur, we let you know which sections you can skip to for further information.

Reviewing the Special Nutritional Needs of People with Type 2 Diabetes

Because most people with type 2 diabetes are overweight, weight management and reduction should be the major consideration. The benefits of weight loss are seen rapidly, even when relatively little weight has been lost. A rapid fall in blood glucose occurs as soon as the energy intake of the diet is reduced. Over time the blood pressure declines and the cholesterol falls. The triglycerides drop and the good cholesterol (HDL) rises. Even a modest reduction of 10 per cent of body weight has a significant positive effect on your coronary artery disease risk.

Unfortunately, your genetic makeup has a significant influence on your ability to lose weight and on the amount of weight you lose. Several studies have shown that people with type 2 diabetes lose less weight than their counterparts without diabetes. This can be disheartening and frustrating — especially when trying to explain not being able to lose weight to less-than-sympathetic workmates, family, friends or (we hate to say) health professionals. But, hang in there — even if weight loss is not possible, weight maintenance is an excellent goal, and you can certainly implement measures to improve the quality of your diet, weight loss or not.

Examining your kilojoule intake

Helen Jacobs, a 46-year-old office worker, was a new patient with type 2 diabetes who came to her endocrinologist because of high blood glucose levels, some blurring of her vision and numbness in her toes. She was 1.65 metres tall and weighed 84.8 kilograms. This gave her a body mass index of 30.9 — putting her in the obese range. (See the section 'Checking your weight' later in this chapter for more on calculating your BMI.) She was taking tablets for her diabetes. Her GP had told her she needed to lose weight, and referred her to her local specialist diabetes dietitian. Helen started on a healthy eating plan, reducing the amount of saturated fat, increasing fibre and reducing the portion size of her meals. Her plan also included increasing her levels of physical activity to offset her sedentary job. She followed her plan and lost 8 kilograms, which she has kept off. Her blood glucose is now in the range of 6.1 to 8.0 mmol/L most of the time. She no longer has blurring of vision, and her toes are beginning to improve. Her endocrinologist has reduced Helen's diabetes medication and she feels much better. Her GP is now looking after her diabetes as the specialist does not need to see her for a year.

No matter how you cut it, your weight is determined by the number of kilojoules you take in, minus the number of kilojoules you use up by exercise. If more kilojoules come in, you gain weight. If fewer kilojoules come in than go out, you lose weight.

The good news is, if you are overweight, you benefit from even a small weight loss. Weight loss

✔ Markedly reduces the risk of developing type 2 diabetes

✔ Prevents the progression of prediabetes (refer to Chapter 5) to type 2 diabetes

✔ Can reverse the failure to respond to drugs for diabetes that develops after responding at first (refer to Chapter 10 for more on medications)

✔ Increases life expectancy in people with type 2 diabetes

✔ Has beneficial effects on high blood pressure and abnormal blood fats

✔ Improves energy levels

✔ Improves mobility

Kilojoule needs are different for different ages, different sexes and different levels of activity — for example, if a woman is pregnant or breastfeeding, she needs more kilojoules. However, a basic principle remains: If a person is trying to lose weight, then reducing the total kilojoules per day can help achieve this. Like Helen, you may do even better if you can increase your level of physical activity — see Chapter 12 for more help in this area.

Try to identify around 2,000 kilojoules that you can remove from your diet per day. By removing this number of kilojoules, you can lose around 0.5 kg per week. The fewer kilojoules you remove, the slower your weight loss will be.

Three basic food groups contain kilojoules: Carbohydrates, proteins and fats. The following sections cover these main groups, highlighting which are the best choices in each group to help you meet your long-term health goals.

Alcohol also contains kilojoules — see the section 'Considering the effect of alcohol' later in this chapter for more.

Considering carbohydrates

Specialists recommend that carbohydrate that's high in fibre and low in fat should contribute between 40 and 50 per cent of your total daily kilojoule intake. An important part of achieving this target is avoiding the sources of carbohydrates that contain lots of kilojoules, but offer little nutritional value.

You probably already have some idea about which carbohydrates only provide 'empty' kilojoules. Just to be clear, here are some examples:

✔ Cakes, biscuits and sweet pastries

✔ Honey and jam

✔ Ice-cream and sweet yoghurt

✔ Lollies and chocolate

✔ Regular soft drinks and cordials

✔ Sugar added to drinks and breakfast cereal

The best carbohydrate choices for you are those that are highest in fibre and lowest in fat — studies have shown that a diet featuring these types of foods can lower blood glucose and cholesterol levels.

Fibre is the part of a food that is not digestible and therefore adds no kilojoules. Fibre is found in all fruits, vegetables and cereal grains, and the more unprocessed the grain (or fruit or vegetable), the higher the fibre content.

Checking the glycaemic index

By avoiding carbohydrates that are high in kilojoules but low in nutritional value, you significantly reduce your intake of sugar (glucose), lowering your blood glucose levels very rapidly. As well as this, choosing foods high in fibre is a good way to satisfy hunger (although not the only way — see the following section on protein for more on this). Foods high in fibre also tend to have a lower glycaemic index.

The glycaemic index (GI) is a measure of how fast a carbohydrate food is digested. Slowly digested carbohydrate foods release their glucose into the bloodstream more slowly, leaving the pancreas more time to provide the right amount of insulin.

The lower the GI of a food, the better, but the quantity eaten is still important. Foods that are excellent sources of carbohydrate but have a low GI include legumes such as lentils, split peas or beans, pasta, grains like barley, basmati rice and some wholegrain breads.

Because carbohydrates such as breads, pasta and breakfasts cereals often make up a large portion of your daily intake, switching to low-GI options in these areas can make a major difference in the overall GI of your diet and so on your blood glucose levels.

You can easily make some simple substitutions in your diet, as shown in Table 11-1. (Also listed in Table 11-1 are some examples of specific brands that produce food with proven low GI. See the section 'Reading and interpreting food labels' later in this chapter for more on using food labels to determine which products are the best to buy.)

Table 11-1	Simple Diet Substitutions
High-GI Food	*Low-GI Food*
Bread (wholemeal or white)	Heavily grained bread (examples include Bürgen varieties and Tip Top 9 Grain)
Processed breakfast cereal	Unrefined cereals like oats or processed low-GI cereals (examples include Guardian and All-Bran cereals)
Most potatoes	Pasta, Carisma potatoes, sweet corn or legumes
Most rice, such as jasmine and arborio	Basmati, Doongara or other low-GI rice
Tropical fruit, such as ripe bananas	Temperate-climate fruits such as apples and plums
Plain biscuits and crackers	Biscuits made with dried fruits or whole grains such as oats

You can't always tell whether a food is low GI just by looking at it — for example, the puffing or flattening of grains that occurs during the production of many breakfast cereals can raise the GI of the food, whereas mixing flour and water, rolling, drying and then cooking it (that's pasta!) will lower the GI. To check a food's GI, consult the GI tables available on various websites — but just make sure the site you're looking at is Australian. The make-up of foods and products can differ significantly between countries, and even foods with the same names can have very different GI ratings in other parts of the world. (See Chapter 24 for the best Australian websites to access.)

Even though a food is low GI, you still might have to avoid it if you're trying to reduce your kilojoule intake — or not eat as much of it as you'd like. Low-GI food can still be high in fat, so make sure you also check food's fat content before assuming it's appropriate. Portion size is also important — even if the food is low GI and low in fat, it doesn't mean that you can eat large portions and still lose weight!

Spreading out your carbohydrate choices

Even carbohydrates with low-GI ratings (see preceding section) can eventually raise your blood glucose levels because carbohydrates (that is, starches and sugars) are made from glucose. Because of this, people often think that they should avoid all carbohydrate foods; however, you need some glucose to provide your brain and muscles with the fuel they need to function well. The key to living more healthily is in knowing how much carbohydrate to consume, and when.

You need to limit the total amount of carbohydrate in your diet and also spread it fairly evenly across the day to maintain healthy blood glucose levels. For most people with type 2 diabetes, the best approach is to have three main meals per day, each containing a moderate amount of carbohydrate, and to have these meals at regular times.

Some people may require snacks in addition to their three main meals per day because of the type of medication they are on. Your expert diabetes dietitian can advise you on the most appropriate spread of carbohydrate across the day for you.

See the section 'Putting it all together: Planning meals' later in this chapter for more on suitable amounts of carbohydrates to eat when wanting to lose weight and stay healthy.

Choosing proteins

Protein is used by the body for growing and repairing tissues. For this reason, it was thought that you could build your own muscle by eating lots of protein (actually, you build up muscle by exercising). Although children and young adults need more protein because they're growing, adults need relatively little protein in order to maintain their current level of muscle.

Protein in your diet comes from chicken, pork, beef, kangaroo, lamb, eggs, milk and other dairy foods, nuts and legumes (or pulses). The protein component of these foods doesn't raise blood glucose levels.

Your choice of protein is still very important because some protein sources are very high in fat (usually saturated fat) whereas some are relatively fat-free. Wherever possible, you should choose lean types of protein foods because in these foods you get more protein than fat, making the energy (or kilojoule) content for these foods lower. For example, having 100 grams of salami on your sandwich will provide you with 1,733 kilojoules just in the salami. By substituting that with 100 grams of lean roast beef, you will get 736 kilojoules (and much less salt!).

Children and young adults should have three or four serves of protein per day; however, for most adults two moderate-sized serves of protein per day are sufficient. As milk, yoghurt and legumes are sources of protein and carbohydrate, they can be included in the diet to satisfy your requirements for both food types.

A certain amount of controversy surrounds the question of how much protein should be in the diet. Most international recommendations state that protein should contribute between 10 and 20 per cent of your total daily kilojoules. However, some studies show that protein is more likely to satisfy your hunger, so a slightly higher percentage of protein in your diet may help your weight-loss efforts.

Rather than focus on strict daily consumption percentages, the most important factor to keep an eye on is the amount of fat that comes with your protein choices. It's okay if the percentage of protein in your diet is a little higher than the recommended 10 to 20 per cent if you select protein with less fat.

We don't recommend that anyone, and especially not children or adolescents, remove all carbohydrate from their diet and replace it with protein foods. You need a balanced diet, not one that is overloaded with one food type or nutrient. For adults, about a quarter of your plate should be covered by the protein part of your meal.

The following lists give you an idea of the fat content of various sources of protein. If you choose your protein from the very lean and lean categories as often as possible, and cut down on some of your carbohydrate intake, you can still achieve your weight loss goals. (In the next section, we explain how to incorporate good fat into your diet.)

Examples of **very lean** meat, fish or substitutes include

- Lean veal, beef, pork or lamb (grilled or baked)
- Legumes (such as soya beans and lentils)
- Lobster, prawns and crab
- Skim/low-fat milk, low-fat yoghurt and cottage cheese
- Skinless white chicken meat or turkey (grilled or baked)
- Tofu or *Quorn* (a vegetarian protein source made from fungi similar to mushrooms)
- White fish or tuna canned in brine or spring water

Lean meat, fish or substitute options include the following:

- An egg
- Bacon (fat-trimmed and grilled)
- Dark chicken meat without skin (grilled or baked)
- Ricotta cheese
- Salmon canned in brine or tuna canned in oil
- Soya beans

Examples of **high-fat** meat or substitutes include

- Cheddar, blue vein, camembert, feta and cream cheeses
- Nuts
- Processed meats, such as sausages, salami, devon and mortadella

See the section 'Putting it all together: Planning meals' later in this chapter for more on incorporating the right sorts of protein choices into your diet.

If you're unsure about the mix of carbohydrates and proteins that's right for you, get in touch with your specialist diabetes dietitian for an individualised assessment.

Monitoring the fat in your diet

Very little disagreement exists among scientists and researchers about the need to limit fat intake! Everyone agrees that you should eat no more than 30 per cent of your diet as fats. As with protein (refer to the preceding section), the type of fat that you eat needs to be considered as well as the quantity.

Dietary fat comes in several forms:

- **Saturated** fat is the kind of fat that mainly comes from animal sources. For example, the streaks of fat in a steak are saturated fat; butter is made up of saturated fat. Bacon, cream, cheese, pastries, cakes, biscuits and chocolate are other examples that contain saturated fat. There are two non-animal sources of saturated fat: Palm oil and coconut milk. Eating a lot of saturated fat increases the blood cholesterol level.

- **Unsaturated** fat comes from vegetable sources such as nuts and seeds. It comes in several forms:

  - Monounsaturated fat doesn't raise cholesterol. Avocado, olive oil, canola oil, olive and canola spreads are examples. The oil in nuts like almonds and peanuts is monounsaturated.

  - Polyunsaturated fat also doesn't raise cholesterol but does cause a reduction in the good or HDL cholesterol. Examples of polyunsaturated fats are soft fats and oils such as sunflower, soybean, sesame oil, oily fish (trout) and sunflower spread.

Although 30 per cent of your total daily kilojoules should come from fat, less than one-third of this amount should come from saturated fats.

Even though the Inuit people indigenous to Greenland, northern Canada and Alaska generally eat far more fat than is recommended, they have a low incidence of heart disease. Their protection against heart disease is created by the presence in their diet of essential fatty acids. These acids are found in fish oils, which the Inuits traditionally consume in large amounts. Essential fatty acids reduce triglycerides, reduce blood pressure and increase the time that it takes for blood to clot, which protects against a blood clot forming in your blood vessels. You can reap the benefits of fish oil by substituting fish for meat two or three times a week.

If you dislike fish — or just can't eat two to three serves of it each week — fish oil capsules are a good substitute. Just make sure when buying the capsules that they contain sufficient quantities of the two active ingredients *eicosapentaenoic acid* (EPA) and *docosahexaenoic acid* (DHA). You should take between 1,200 milligrams and 3,000 milligrams of a combination of these active ingredients each day. To make it easier, many formulations of fish oil are now concentrated, meaning you only need to take one or two capsules per day to reach the 1,200 milligrams per day target.

Putting it all together: Planning meals

A balanced diet contains regular amounts of carbohydrates, proteins and fats with sufficient variety to provide you with all the vitamins and minerals you require for health. To give you an idea of the types and quantities of foods you should aim to be eating, the following lists your daily targets, broken into carbohydrates, proteins, fats and your vitamin- and mineral-rich essentials.

Meals should be spread across the day. Although children are more likely to need snacks because their stomachs are small and they can't always eat enough at meal times to satisfy their nutritional requirements, only some adults require regular snacks in addition to their three main meals.

When selecting carbohydrates, keep in mind the following:

- This group includes bread, potato, rice and other grains, pasta, fruit, breakfast cereals, milk and yoghurt.

- Food from this group should provide between 40 and 50 per cent of your energy needs for the day. This equates to two to three serves of carbohydrate at each meal for a small person or someone trying to lose weight or up to twice this much for a lean, large and/or active person.

- Two to three serves of carbohydrate equates to covering about a quarter of your plate with these foods.

✔ One serve of carbohydrates is approximately equal to a slice of bread, a piece of fruit, third of a cup of cooked rice, half a cup of grains, cereals, starchy vegetables or cooked pasta, 200 grams of plain yoghurt, or 300 millilitres of milk.

✔ You should aim to choose low-fat, high-fibre options.

✔ You should try to have two pieces of fruit each day.

The following factors are important when considering protein food choices:

✔ This group includes meat, chicken, fish, eggs, dairy foods, nuts and legumes.

✔ Food from this group should make up between 10 and 20 per cent of an adult's diet. This equates to two moderate-sized serves per day for an adult.

✔ One small serve of protein is approximately equal to 90 grams of meat or chicken, 150 grams of fish, two large eggs, 40 grams of cheese, 30 grams of nuts or half a cup of cooked legumes.

✔ You should aim to choose low-fat varieties.

✔ You should cook and prepare these foods with as little added fat (and salt) as possible.

To ensure they eat enough protein, vegetarians should include nuts, legumes and/or dairy foods in their diets each day. Those who also avoid dairy foods should also have an extra serve of protein to ensure their daily requirements are met, as the density of the protein in nuts and legumes is not as high as in animal sources. Vegetable sources of protein should be eaten with grains to ensure the protein provided in the meal contains all the essential amino acids for health.

Keep in mind the following when looking at fats in your food choices:

✔ This group includes butter, margarine, oils, mayonnaise, salad dressings, cream and sour cream.

✔ Fat should only make up approximately 30 per cent of your diet.

✔ Your first choice from the fat options should be polyunsaturated or monounsaturated fats, such as margarine and oils.

✔ Most people don't need more than one tablespoon of added unsaturated fats (such as vegetable margarines and oils) each day, because their carbohydrate and protein choices will already contain some fats as well.

✔ When buying cooking oils, always choose oils where the source of the oil (such as olive, canola, sunflower or peanut) is labelled.

✔ You shouldn't be tempted to cut out fat altogether! The human body needs essential fatty acids and fat-soluble vitamins to function well, and these are provided by these fats.

As a bit of a bonus, you also get to choose from what we call *free foods*. The name says it all, really — these are foods that contain few carbohydrates, fats or proteins, but provide fibre and essential vitamins and minerals to our daily diet. You can go ahead and eat these foods freely to add bulk and interest to your diet!

Keep in mind the following when selecting free foods:

✔ Options in this group include all vegetables (except potato, sweet potato and sweet corn), lemons, grapefruit, passionfruit and rhubarb.

✔ At mealtimes, you want half your plate covered by free foods such as vegetables or salad.

✔ Low-kilojoule foods are also included in this group, such as mustard, pickles, chutney, herbs and spices, Vegemite and oil-free dressings.

Losing Weight with Type 2 Diabetes

If you have type 2 diabetes and are overweight or obese, the health benefits of losing even a small amount of weight are large. The following sections help you check your weight, so you know where you are right now, and offer guidance to the various weight-loss methods available.

Checking your weight

To give you a general idea of how much you ought to weigh, you can use a formula called the *body mass index* (BMI), which relates your weight to your height — so if you are shorter than someone who weighs the same as you, you will have the higher BMI. A person with a BMI under 20 is considered underweight. A person with a BMI from 20 to 25 is a normal weight. A person with a BMI from 25.1 to 29.9 is overweight, and a person with a BMI of 30 or over is obese. By this definition, around 66 per cent of people in Australia are overweight or obese.

You cannot step on a scale and get a reading of your BMI, but you can get your weight. This is one of the easiest measurements in medicine.

To work out your BMI, take your weight (in kilograms) and divide it by your height (in metres) squared. For example, say you weigh 82 kilograms and are 1.69 metres tall. Your BMI is 82 divided by 2.8561 (1.69 squared), or 28.7 — putting you in the overweight range.

Maintaining a BMI as close as possible to the normal range makes controlling your diabetes and blood pressure easier.

Reducing your weight

Weight reduction is difficult for many reasons. In our experience, most people do very well initially but tend to return to old habits because it's so hard to keep on track all the time. Evidence suggests that this tendency to regain weight is built into the human brain. When fat tissue is decreased or even increased, a central control system in the brain acts to restore the fat to the previous level. If liposuction is done, for example, the remaining cells swell up to hold more fat.

Still, losing weight and keeping it off is possible. It is just very difficult and requires lifelong effort.

In Chapter 12, we discuss the value of exercise in a weight loss program. At this point, you need to realise that successful maintenance of weight loss requires a willingness to make exercise a part of your daily life. If, for some reason, you cannot move your legs to exercise, you can get a satisfactory workout using your upper body alone. A recent study showed that 92 per cent of the people who maintained weight loss were exercising regularly, while only 34 per cent of those who regained their weight continued to exercise.

Checking out types of diets

The endless number of diets that are around certainly suggest that no one method is any better than all the others. Some are fairly drastic in the degree to which they cut kilojoules, and weight loss is fairly rapid. However, when you come off one of these quick weight loss diets, more often than not you quickly put back on all the weight you lost.

Check with your GP or diabetes care team if you're planning to try a quick weight loss diet because your diabetes medications may need to be changed.

Among the more drastic diets are the following:

✔ **Very low kilojoule diets:** On a daily basis, these diets provide 1,600 to 3,300 kilojoules with supplemental vitamins and minerals. They're safe for people with diabetes when supervised by a diabetes dietitian or doctor. They can be used when you need rapid weight loss, such as before an operation. They result in rapid initial weight loss with a fall in the need for medication. Weight restoration commonly occurs, but will depend on what dietary pattern and exercise level you follow afterwards.

These diets are not easy to follow as you are often required to replace proper meals with a drink or bar. This makes them rather socially unacceptable — and not that attractive when family and friends around you are all eating 'proper' food! However, they can be very useful for some people — just check with your diabetes dietitian or GP first if you think this kind of diet may be a suitable approach for you.

✔ **Very high protein diets:** Food is limited to animal protein sources in an effort to maintain body protein, meaning the diet contains very little carbohydrate. A supplement with a full complement of vitamins and minerals should be taken when following these diets. Patients often complain of tiredness, constipation and bad breath. Weight is regained rapidly when the diet is discontinued. This diet is not balanced and we don't recommend it for more than a few weeks.

✔ **Fasts:** A *fast* means giving up all food for a period of time and taking only water and vitamins and minerals. A fast is such a drastic change from normal eating habits that people don't remain on the fast for very long, and the weight lost is usually quickly regained. These diets can be dangerous and should be avoided.

Several diets are associated with large organisations that often require you to purchase only their foods. The support given by some of these organisations seems to be extremely helpful in weight loss maintenance. In addition, the slower loss of weight and the similarity of the diet to normal eating habits seem to result in a greater tendency to stay with the program and keep the weight off. However, people who go on a weight loss program need to understand that they will regain the weight if they don't make permanent changes to their lifestyle.

As organisations and groups offering weight loss programs proliferated, some of them far from reputable, the need to regulate the weight loss industry arose. The Weight Management Code Administration Council of Australia administers a code of practice for the industry. The code of practice ensures truthful advertising with authentic success stories, accurate information (including complete cost proposals) and an overall reliable and safe service. An organisation can become a member of the council and is then bound by the code.

When choosing a weight loss program, check that the service provider is a member of the Weight Management Code Administration Council of Australia, and so is bound by its code of practice.

The leading contenders in Australia for this type of diet are

- **Jenny Craig:** This organisation provides the food that you eat, which you pay for. Nutritional information about the food is available and the regularity of the provided meals can be helpful. Some information on behaviour modification is offered and participants have access to a trained advisor as required. A letter from your doctor may be required prior to starting the program.

- **Lite n' Easy:** This organisation provides the food that you eat, which you pay for. Some information on behaviour modification is offered in the form of online articles and tip sheets. The nutritional value of the meals is easily available and this can help people with diabetes achieve a regularity they can benefit from.

- **Weight Watchers:** This organisation emphasises slow weight loss, exercise and behaviour modification. You are charged for weekly attendance at meetings, which are held all over the world. Weight Watchers food products are available in the supermarket; however, you are not required to purchase any of these products. The new Weight Watchers ProPoints program may not be especially helpful to someone with diabetes as it's not specifically designed for those with diabetes; however, the information provided can be adapted to your needs with help from a specialist diabetes dietitian.

The costs of the programs covered in the preceding list are prohibitive for some people, so working with a specialist diabetes dietitian may be a better option for you. Dietitian services can be accessed free of charge through your state or territory health department, or visits to a private dietitian can be subsidised by Medicare. (Government-funded access to dietitians requires a referral from a GP.)

Taking medications

Because most people with type 2 diabetes are struggling with their weight and their glucose control improves with weight loss, the search for weight-lowering drugs has been enthusiastic, to say the least.

The most commonly used weight loss medication in the Australia is orlistat, which is marketed as Xenical. Orlistat is a *gastrointestinal lipase inhibitor*, which means that it reduces the absorption of fat in the diet. If you eat too much fat, it remains in the intestine, reaches the stool, and can cause flatulence, oily bowel movements and even bowel incontinence. Because of these side effects, some people stop taking the drug. However, such side effects disappear when the fat content of the diet is sufficiently low. This is how it works — it forces you to maintain your low-fat (and therefore low-kilojoule) diet! Otherwise, the consequences can be unpleasant, to say the least.

In a study specifically for people with diabetes, a group using orlistat lost much more weight than a non-orlistat group. The orlistat users were able to reduce their blood glucose, their haemoglobin A1c and their need for oral sulphonylurea medication, as well as their elevated cholesterol levels. Very few of the orlistat-takers stopped taking the drug and left the study because of intestinal or bowel problems. Orlistat could be a major new weapon against the obesity that worsens the effects of diabetes and threatens coronary artery disease. However, its use may be limited by the fact that it is very expensive. You can buy orlistat over the counter at pharmacies. (Refer to Chapter 10 for more on medications for weight loss.)

The search for other suitable weight loss drugs continues but further options remain elusive. Unfortunately, unintended side effects are a problem and several weight loss drugs have appeared on the market only to be removed several years later when problems occur. This is disappointing for both patient and doctor!

Undergoing surgery

Surgery for weight reduction is currently used in the more severe cases of obesity. Surgery can have impressive effects such as correction of high glucose levels and reduction or discontinuation of glucose-lowering drugs. Some of the reasons for considering surgical procedures to treat obesity are as follows:

- ✔ You have a BMI that is greater than 35.

- ✔ You have an obesity-related physical problem limiting your ability to walk.

- ✔ You have an obesity-related health problem like diabetes.

- ✔ You have been unable to lose the excess weight with traditional programs involving diet, exercise, behaviour modification and medication.

Three main surgical procedures are carried out to help in the management of severe obesity. The first involves the placement of an adjustable band, known as a *lap band*, around the stomach to reduce its size. Because your stomach is smaller, you feel full despite eating less and therefore lose weight. The band is placed through a small hole in your abdomen, which is a much less invasive procedure than the other two alternatives (gastric bypass or gastric sleeve surgery). To adjust the band, saline solution can be added to or removed from a small reservoir under the skin, which causes the band to expand or deflate, altering the size of your stomach and therefore the amount of food that can be consumed. In the early days a small amount of fluid is placed in the band, but as the weight loss slows over time the band can be tightened.

Studies have shown that by the end of the first year, people who had undergone lap band surgery had lost half of their excess weight. After two years, the average BMI had come down from 45 to 31, with a weight loss of nearly 60 per cent of the excess weight. Noticeable improvements have been seen in people with type 2 diabetes, hypertension and high cholesterol.

Some of the problems that may occur when a lap band is in place include

- ✔ Prolapse of the stomach through the band, which requires replacement of the band.

- ✔ Rupture of the reservoir tubing, which requires a minor procedure to repair.

- ✔ Erosion of the band into the stomach wall, which has occurred in a small number of cases and requires replacement of the band.

- ✔ Gallstones, which have not caused symptoms previously, can become more active.

The second surgical procedure is the *gastric bypass operation*, where the stomach is stapled to create a small pouch. A section of the small intestine is attached to the pouch so food passes through very little of the small intestine, reducing kilojoule and nutrient absorption. Because the pouch is small, you tend to eat less. Because much of the digestive system is bypassed you also absorb fewer kilojoules. Not only is a good quality multivitamin required for life, but you will also need to take supplements of calcium and iron. The usual loss of weight is two-thirds of the excess in two years.

Some of the problems of gastric bypass include:

- ✔ The pouch may stretch.

- ✔ The staple line can break down.

- ✔ Malabsorption of iron and calcium may occur.

- ✔ Anaemia may occur from lack of vitamin B12.

- ✔ The *dumping syndrome* may occur. In this condition, stomach contents move too fast into the small intestine, provoking a lot of insulin with resultant hypoglycaemia.

The third surgical procedure is known as the *gastric sleeve*. This procedure is similar to the gastric bypass; however, the shape of the remaining stomach is slightly larger and more elongated. In this procedure, the early part of the small intestine is bypassed, causing your body to forgo absorption of some fats, vitamins and minerals. As with a gastric bypass, a good quality multivitamin is required for life. Similar problems to those that can occur with a gastric bypass (included in the preceding list) can also occur.

Both the gastric bypass and the gastric sleeve are operations that are not reversible and both can have a serious impact on your health and lifestyle. Make sure you talk with your GP and diabetes care team and consider all your options before deciding on surgery.

When you have a surgical procedure as treatment for obesity, you must be willing to commit to lifelong medical and dietetic follow-up. You must undertake a program of diet and exercise, and change your behaviour towards food. You must also be determined to lose the weight and keep it off. Without these changes, the success of these procedures can be very limited. These surgical procedures are not available on Medicare, but may be covered by your private health fund.

If you wish to undergo any of the procedures covered in this section, discuss it with your GP and be referred to an experienced practitioner who works within a multidisciplinary health team. This will ensure the best success possible.

Modifying behaviour

Diet and exercise must be accompanied by changes in behaviour with respect to food. Adjusting eating behaviour makes the diet easier to stick to; some of the best techniques include the following:

- At the supermarket, buy from a list, carry only enough money for the food on that list (and no cards), and avoid aisles containing high-kilojoule treat foods such as lollies.
- Do not conscientiously clean your plate.
- Eat according to a schedule to avoid eating between meals.
- Eat all your meals at the table.
- Plate food in the kitchen.
- Set realistic goals for weight loss.
- Slow down the rate at which you eat and make the meal last.
- Turn off the TV.
- When eating out, be careful of salad dressing, alcohol and bread.

You can incorporate one technique into your life each week (or whatever period it takes) until you feel you have mastered it and have added it to your eating style. Then go on and adopt another technique.

As you go about this difficult task of losing weight and keeping it off, remember to seek the help of those around you. A loving partner or friend provides great help through the roughest days.

See Chapter 13 for more help on increasing your motivation to make lifestyle changes and maintaining those changes for life.

Substituting sweeteners (kilojoule-containing and artificial)

A vast effort has been made to produce a compound that could add the pleasure of sweetness without the liabilities of sugar. If you can reduce your kilojoule intake or your glucose response by using a sweetener, there is an advantage. Sweeteners are divided into those that contain kilojoules and those that do not.

Among the kilojoule-containing sweeteners are

- **Fructose, found in fruits and berries:** Fructose is actually sweeter than table sugar (sucrose). The sweetener is absorbed more slowly from the intestine than glucose, so it raises the blood glucose more slowly.

- **Sorbitol and mannitol, sugar alcohols occurring in plants:** Sorbitol and mannitol are half as sweet as table sugar and still have some effect on blood glucose.

- **Xylitol, found in strawberries and raspberries:** Xylitol is very similar to fructose in terms of sweetness. Slowly taken up from the intestine so that it causes little change in blood glucose, xylitol doesn't cause tooth decay as often as the other nutritive sweeteners.

For people with type 2 diabetes, it's best to avoid the sweeteners included in the preceding list because of their high energy intake. (For those with type 1 diabetes, if you use these sweeteners, you need to include them in your calculations of the total carbohydrate in your meal; see the section 'Counting carbohydrates' later in this chapter for more.)

The non-nutritive or artificial sweeteners are often much sweeter than table sugar. Therefore, much less of them is required to achieve the same level of sweetness as sugar. They contain minimal kilojoules and so are the sweeteners of choice. The current artificial sweeteners include

- **Aspartame (Hermasetas Gold and Equal):** This sweetener is more expensive than saccharin, but people seem to prefer its taste. Aspartame is 150 to 200 times sweeter than sucrose.

- **Cyclamate:** Cyclamate is not used as a table sweetener, and can be found in some drinks, such as diet cordial, mixed with saccharin. Cyclamate is 30 times as sweet as sucrose.

- **Saccharin (Sugarella and Sugarine):** Saccharin is 300 to 400 times sweeter than sucrose, and is rapidly excreted unchanged in the urine.

✔ **Sucralose (Splenda):** The sweetener sucralose is 600 times sweeter than sucrose. It's available in tablets and powder form and is found in some diet drinks and diet yoghurts.

✔ **Stevia (PureVia):** Although it has been available overseas for many years, stevia is the newest non-nutritive sweetener on the market in Australia. It is made from a plant of South American origin and is up to 300 times sweeter than sucrose. It is available for use as a table sweetener.

Other artificial sweeteners approved for use in Australia include acesulphame-K, alitame and thaumatin. These are usually mixed with the other sweeteners and are in few Australian foods.

Kilojoule-containing (or nutritive) sweeteners are best avoided — the non-nutritive or artificial sweeteners will provide the sweet taste but almost none of the extra energy that you don't need when trying to lose weight. Also, non-nutritive sweeteners won't raise your blood glucose levels like kilojoule-containing sweeteners will!

Useful foods and drinks containing artificial sweeteners are

✔ 'Diet' or 'Zero' soft drinks

✔ Low-joule jelly and cordial

✔ Reduced-sugar yoghurt

✔ 'Sugar-free' lollies and chewing gum

If you wish to replace sugar in recipes requiring heating (such as baking or boiling), the best substitutes are sucralose and stevia. These artificial sweeteners remain stable during cooking and will most often give you the best texture and taste. However, replacing all the sugar in a recipe with either of these sweeteners will not always result in the same look or texture you may be used to. If this is the case, try replacing half or two-thirds of the sugar with the artificial sweetener, for a dish that both tastes and 'feels' good!

As yet, no sugar-free chocolate is available in Australia — enjoy a small serve of the real thing instead!

Reading and interpreting food labels

Most food products in Australia have a nutrition information panel (NIP). The NIP allows you to compare information to determine healthier products. You can use the panels to compare the fat, saturated fat, fibre and sodium levels of similar products.

To compare products effectively, look at the amounts in the 100-gram column, rather than the serving-size column. That way, you're comparing like with like.

As a rough guide, aim for:

✔ Total fat less than 10 grams per 100 grams; for milk and yoghurt, aim for less than 2 grams of fat per 100 grams.

✔ Saturated fat as low as possible; ideally, saturated fat should be less than 3 grams per 100 grams.

✔ Products with the highest fibre; look for cereals greater than 6 grams of fibre per 100 grams and bread greater than 5 grams of fibre per 100 grams.

✔ Cereals with less than 400 milligrams of sodium per 100 grams and bread with less than 450 milligrams per 100 grams. A low-sodium product contains less than 120 milligrams of sodium per 100 grams.

Figure 11-1 shows an example of a NIP, with the areas you should pay most attention to shaded in grey.

Figure 11-1	**Example Food Label**	

Nutrition Information
Servings per package: 18
Serving size: 33 grams (2 biscuits)

	Per Serving	Per 100 Grams
Energy (kJ)	492 kJ	1490 kJ
(Cal)	118 Cal	356 Cal
Protein (g)	4.1 g	12.4 g
Fat – Total (g)	0.5 g	1.4 g
– Saturated fat (g)	0.1 g	0.3 g
Carbohydrate – Total (g)	22.1 g	67 g
– Sugars (g)	1.1 g	3.3 g
Dietary fibre (g)	3.6 g	11.0 g
Sodium (mg)	96 mg	290 mg

Reviewing the Special Nutritional Needs of People with Type 1 Diabetes

Unlike a person with type 2 diabetes, a person with type 1 doesn't necessarily need to lose weight — they more often have other important issues about food to consider! At diagnosis, most people with type 1 diabetes have lost significant amounts of weight and need to regain this to get back to their usual healthy selves.

A person with type 1 diabetes takes insulin to control the blood glucose levels that arise after eating food containing carbohydrate. It is very difficult with injected insulin to match the human pancreas in the way that it releases insulin just when the food is entering the bloodstream so that the glucose remains exactly between healthy levels of 4 and 8 mmol/L.

However, it is possible to try to mimic the actions of the pancreas by taking two different types of insulin, one that acts soon after the injection and has a brief period of activity, and a second kind of insulin that acts more slowly and lasts longer. The rapid-acting insulin is meant to cover the carbohydrate food eaten at meals, while the slower acting insulin covers the rest of the time, particularly overnight when a lot of circumstances tend to raise the blood glucose. (Refer to Chapter 10 for more on the different kinds of insulin, and when and how they can be taken or injected.)

To predict the amount of rapid-acting insulin you require for a meal if you have type 1 diabetes, you need to estimate the amount of carbohydrate in the meal and give a matching amount of insulin. Does this sound complex?! Well, it takes a little while to master, but the following sections show you how, as well as providing some tips on how much fat should be incorporated into your diet, what you should take into account if you are trying to lose weight, and the special diet considerations for children and teens with type 1 diabetes.

Counting carbohydrates

Carbohydrates include both starchy and sugary foods. Carbohydrates are broken down into glucose in your intestinal tract to provide your body with energy. Some of the common sources of carbohydrate are bread, potatoes, grains and fruit.

Before you develop diabetes, your pancreas produces just the right amount of insulin to cover the rise in blood glucose after carbohydrates are consumed. After type 1 diabetes develops, the pancreas can no longer perform this role, so people with type 1 diabetes needs to learn how to 'think like a pancreas' and make their insulin dose decisions each time they eat based on the amount of carbohydrate they eat.

Throughout most of Australia, 15 grams of carbohydrate is used as a reference amount for counting the carbohydrate in food. This amount is called an *exchange*. Each exchange of carbohydrate you eat is matched by a certain amount of rapid-acting insulin.

Some states in Australia have decided to take on the United Kingdom's carbohydrate exchange measurement of 10 grams of carbohydrate (which they call a portion). If this system is used where you live, the quantities below will be slightly different, but the principles of matching insulin are the same.

Examples of one carbohydrate exchange (15 grams of carbohydrate) include the following:

- One slice of white, wholemeal or wholegrain bread
- One average-sized piece of fruit
- One medium potato
- Half a cup of mashed potato/sweet corn/sweet potato/peas
- Half a cup of cooked pasta
- One-third of a cup of cooked rice
- 300 millilitres of full cream/skim/low-fat milk or soy milk
- 200-gram tub of plain or reduced-sugar yoghurt
- Two plain sweet biscuits
- Two large crackers (such as Ryvita) or four small crackers (such as Vita-Weats)

The amount of insulin you need to inject for each carbohydrate exchange will depend on many different factors, including your age, body size and sensitivity to insulin. A person with type 1 diabetes may have a ratio anywhere between approximately half a unit and five units of insulin per one carbohydrate exchange.

Your specialist diabetes dietitian will calculate your individual *insulin to carbohydrate ratio* (how much insulin you require to match each exchange of carbohydrate). To determine your ratio, your dietitian will ask you to provide a detailed food diary and take extra finger-prick blood glucose tests.

Once you know your insulin to carbohydrate ratio, you have the freedom to eat any type of carbohydrate. You just have to 'know your carbs' and then put the right amount of insulin with the amount you eat. Your dietitian will help you to learn how to determine the carbohydrate content of the foods you eat. This includes checking the information written on the labels of foods you buy.

To work out carbohydrate exchanges from a food label, use the per serving column. Compare the serving size listed (for example, two biscuits) to the amount of the food you are going to eat. If you're eating the recommended serving size, look at the total carbohydrate per serving (not the sugar) and divide by 15. For example, if each serve contains 22.1 grams total carbohydrate, this equals 1.5 exchanges (22.1 divided by 15). If you're eating more or less than the suggested serving size, you'll need to adjust your calculations accordingly.

Like all Australians, all people with type 1 diabetes should follow a healthy diet — that is, a diet that's not too high in fat and sugar, contains plenty of fibre and minimises excessive weight gain. However, we are realistic enough to understand that this is not always possible all of the time! No-one is perfect and we would simply encourage you to do your best. Support from your diabetes care team is available to help you learn more about healthy carbohydrate choices and be supported in your efforts to look after yourself. (Refer to the section 'Considering carbohydrates' earlier in this chapter for more on the best carbohydrate options.)

While you should always try to inject your rapid-acting insulin before you eat, there are times when you may be unsure how much carbohydrate will be in your meal — for example, when you eat out at a restaurant and you have several courses. In these situations you can wait until after the meal, counting carbohydrate exchanges as you go, and inject once you've finished eating. This tactic is also useful for children when they're going to parties or being a bit 'fussy' about what they will eat.

Does fat matter?

Even though weight problems and obesity are associated more with people with type 2, rather than type 1, diabetes, dietary fat matters for all Australians! Dietary fat, especially saturated fat found in animal foods, is the most potent increaser of blood cholesterol levels. Fat also has twice the energy value gram for gram as carbohydrate and protein, making it an easy way to consume excess kilojoules. Because people with type 1 diabetes are also at increased risk for coronary artery disease, you need to watch your cholesterol levels (and blood pressure!) and ensure they stay in the target range — and a low-fat diet can help.

It's okay to treat yourself (or your children) to high-fat foods once in a while — just make sure they're not the predominant part of your diet. Even young people with type 1 diabetes who are a healthy weight should be careful about how much and what type of fat they consume.

Refer to the section 'Monitoring the fat in your diet' earlier in this chapter for more on good and bad fats; refer to the section 'Putting it all together: Planning meals' earlier in this chapter for more on planning your daily intake of different kinds of foods.

Some protein choices are very high in fat, and usually saturated fat, so it's best to choose very lean and lean types of protein foods — from both animal and non-animal sources — whenever possible. Refer to the section 'Choosing proteins' earlier in this chapter for more on the best protein choices, as well as how many servings of protein you should be having per day.

Weight loss

As they get older, some people with type 1 diabetes may also find themselves carrying extra weight, which may be detrimental to their overall health. In the past, when people with type 1 diabetes reduced their total kilojoule intake in an attempt to lose weight, they often became hypoglycaemic, because their insulin doses were rarely adjusted to match the reduced intake. Now, with the knowledge people have gained from learning to count carbohydrate and adjust their own insulin doses, people with type 1 diabetes can lose weight more easily and without the worry of repeated and troublesome hypoglycaemia.

Coping with eating disorders and diabetes

You can't be too rich or too thin. How much damage has this statement done to society, especially the last part about being thin? Young people, particularly girls, are fixated with their body weight. When this preoccupation becomes too great, it can result in an eating disorder. The young girl (and young boys, about a tenth as often) will either starve herself and exercise excessively or eat a great deal and then induce vomiting and/or take laxatives and fluid tablets. The one who starves herself has *anorexia nervosa*, while the one who binges and purges has *bulimia nervosa*. By themselves, these conditions can result in severe illness and even death when carried to extremes. When combined with diabetes, there is very great danger to their health.

Anorexia is commonly found in middle- and upper-class girls, who have a distorted body image and are fearful of weight gain. Their parents are usually very concerned with slimness. In Australia, the prevalence is estimated to be as high as one in 100 girls. The girls may appear unusually thin and do not menstruate. These girls are in a constant state of starvation and suffer from such severe malnutrition that they sometimes die from it.

When anorexic young women suffer from diabetes, their condition is just like that of people with type 1 diabetes before the availability of insulin. They lose a lot of body musculature once the fat is gone, and also have very low blood glucose levels, so little or no insulin is required. Such young women develop heart problems and have low blood pressure and low body temperature.

The girl with severe anorexia may require intravenous feeding until she is stabilised. Once the life-threatening starvation is under control, it is possible to achieve better blood glucose control with help from the patient and a counsellor who can help her to understand her distorted body image. If there is clinical depression, antidepressant medication may be necessary.

Bulimia involves eating large quantities of easily digested food and then purging it by vomiting and taking laxatives or fluid tablets. These people are not as severely thin as those with anorexia. Their background is similar to those with anorexia. In Australia 6 per cent of university-aged females are diagnosed with bulimia, but it is thought that between 20 and 40 per cent of this age group have binge-eating disorders. Because their weight is closer to normal, they usually menstruate normally.

Girls with bulimia are more likely to go on to obesity in adulthood and are harder to treat. They actually do not do as well with treatment as those with anorexia. They end up with more psychiatric problems later in life.

The food intake of bulimic girls is extremely variable but less severe than that of those with anorexia.

Both anorexia and bulimia make controlling blood glucose difficult but one other activity makes managing diabetes difficult. Some women and men skip insulin injections in order to lose weight. Weight will be lost as the body turns to fat for fuel because glucose can't be used (refer to Chapter 2). Again, loss of muscle mass occurs and the blood glucose rises very high. Of course, skipping insulin and the resulting high glucose levels will increase the risk of developing the complications of diabetes.

If you would like to know more about anorexia and bulimia, eating-disorder associations are found in most capital cities around Australia. These organisations provide publications and websites with information on disorders and frequently asked questions, local support groups and telephone help lines and email discussion lists. The Butterfly Foundation (www.thebutterflyfoundation.org.au) has information about and links to services all across Australia.

To lose weight, you need to reduce your energy intake (food) and increase your energy output (exercise). Your insulin dose will need to be adjusted around these changes. If you require help with this, speak to your diabetes care team.

For more information on weight loss, refer to the section 'Reducing your weight' earlier in this chapter.

Children and teens

The insulin-to-carbohydrate ratio approach can be also used for children and teenagers with type 1 diabetes (refer to the section 'Counting carbohydrates' earlier in this chapter for more on this approach). With younger children, mums, dads and carers will need to be responsible for ensuring the correct amounts of insulin are given. However, by the time children are hitting high school, these skills can be passed on and the kids encouraged to make decisions about food and insulin doses for themselves.

Children and teenagers don't need to have a 'perfect' diet all of the time — being a kid or a teenager with type 1 diabetes is sometimes not much fun as it is. The main aim is to establish and maintain healthy growth and development with a well-balanced diet that is acceptable in all social situations and that should prevent excess weight gain and any complications of diabetes.

Living with coeliac disease and type 1 diabetes

Coeliac disease is an autoimmune condition where the lining of the small intestine is damaged due to an intolerance to a protein in food called gluten. If left untreated, the condition can lead to malabsorption of nutrients, difficulty managing blood glucose levels, diarrhoea, constipation, flatulence, abdominal pain, nausea, bloating, tiredness, anaemia, skin rashes, infertility, recurring miscarriages and osteoporosis. Approximately 10 per cent of people with type 1 diabetes also have coeliac disease. Because symptoms of the condition can be slow to emerge or hard to identify, if you have type 1 diabetes your doctor should arrange regular blood tests for you to ensure diagnosis is made promptly.

Treatment of coeliac disease requires life-long avoidance of gluten. Gluten is found in wheat, rye, oats, triticale and barley, so people diagnosed with the condition must avoid all foods which are made with these ingredients. This is a dietary restriction that can be difficult to follow; however, help is available from the Coeliac Society in your state and from dietitians with expertise in the condition. Gluten-free foods are also becoming more widely available in supermarkets, specialty shops and online.

For the website details for the Coeliac Society in your state, see Chapter 24. For more help and tips on living with coeliac disease and gluten intolerance, check out *Living Gluten-Free For Dummies*, Australian Edition, by Danna Korn and Margaret Clough (Wiley Publishing Australia Pty Ltd).

By allowing children to eat a less restrictive diet (as long as they inject the correct doses of insulin), some people feared the insulin-to-carbohydrate-ratio approach would lead to excess weight gain. However, at least one scientific study has shown the opposite. By allowing children to be flexible in the timing and quantity of food eaten, most maintained their healthy weight or lost weight!

See Chapter 16 for a more detailed discussion of the specific considerations for children and teenagers with diabetes.

Reviewing General Nutritional Needs of All People with Diabetes

Some general nutritional needs should be considered regardless of whether you have type 1 or type 2 diabetes. The following sections cover tips to ensure you have an adequate intake of vitamins, minerals and water in your diet, and also look at the effect of alcohol.

Getting enough vitamins, minerals and water

Your diet must contain sufficient vitamins and minerals for good health, but the amount you need may be less than you think. If you eat a balanced diet that comes from the various food groups, you generally get enough vitamins for your daily needs. Table 11-2 lists the vitamins and their food sources.

Table 11-2	Vitamins You Need	
Vitamin	*Function*	*Food Source*
Vitamin A	Needed for growth and development, immune function, bones and healthy skin; helps with night vision	Liver, eggs, oily fish, dairy products, orange and green vegetables and orange fruits
Vitamin B1 (thiamine)	Converts carbohydrate into energy	Wholegrain cereals, meat, fish, nuts, yeast extract

(continued)

Table 11-2 *(continued)*

Vitamin B2 (riboflavin)	Needed to release energy from food	Milk, cheese, fish, almonds, eggs, green vegetables and fortified cereals
Vitamin B6 (pyridoxine), pantothenic acid and biotin	Needed for growth, normal brain and nerve function	Bananas, potatoes, wholegrain cereals, meat, fish and nuts
Vitamin B12	Keeps the red blood cells and the nervous system healthy	Animal foods only; for example, meat, seafood, eggs
Folic acid	Keeps the red blood cells and the nervous system healthy	Liver, fortified breakfast cereals, green leafy vegetables and yeast extract
Niacin	Helps release energy	Meat, chicken, fish, nuts, legumes and wholegrain products
Vitamin C	Helps maintain supportive tissues	Fruit and some vegetables; for example, tomatoes and capsicum
Vitamin D	Helps with absorption of calcium	Oily fish, egg yolk and fortified milk and margarines; also made in the skin when exposed to sunlight, although this process declines as you age
Vitamin E	Helps maintain cells	Vegetable oils, nuts, seeds and wholegrain cereals
Vitamin K	Needed for proper clotting of the blood	Green leafy vegetables; also made by bacteria in your intestine

As you look through the vitamins in Table 11-2, you can see that most of them are easily available in the foods you eat every day. (In certain situations, such as during pregnancy, you may need to take a vitamin or mineral supplement to ensure that you are getting enough every day.)

As far as vitamins are concerned, the proof just doesn't exist that large amounts of them are beneficial. In some cases, they may be harmful. We do not recommend that you take megadoses of vitamins.

Minerals are also key ingredients of a healthy diet. Most are needed in tiny amounts, which, with a few exceptions, are easily consumed from a balanced diet. These essential minerals are as follows:

- ✔ **Calcium, phosphorous and magnesium build bones and teeth:** Milk and other dairy products provide plenty of these minerals, but evidence suggests that people aren't getting enough calcium. It is recommended that young children get 500 to 700 milligrams of calcium every day, adolescents get 1,000 to 1,300 milligrams each day and adults get 1,000 milligrams. Women over 50 years and men over 70 years are recommended to have 1,300 milligrams each day. Pregnant women and breastfeeding mothers should have 1,000 milligrams, particularly in the final three months of the pregnancy and throughout the breastfeeding period.

- ✔ **Iodine is essential for production of thyroid hormones:** Iodine is often added to salt in order to ensure that people get enough of it. In many areas of the world where iodine is not found in the soil, people suffer from very large thyroid glands known as *goitres*.

- ✔ **Iron is essential for red blood cells:** Iron is obtained from red meat and iron-fortified breakfast cereals. Green leafy vegetables provide small amounts of iron; however, it is not in a form that's easily absorbed by the body. A menstruating woman loses iron each month and may need to supplement her food with a tablet. Vegetarians and pregnant or breastfeeding mothers may also require a supplement.

- ✔ **Sodium regulates body water:** You need only about 300 milligrams a day but may take in 20 to 40 times that much, which probably explains a lot of the high blood pressure in Australia. Don't add salt to your food because it already has plenty in it — and you'll enjoy the taste a lot more without it.

- ✔ **Chromium is needed in tiny amounts:** No scientific evidence shows that chromium is especially helpful to the person with diabetes in controlling the blood glucose, despite reams of articles in health food magazines to the contrary.

- ✔ Various other minerals, like **chlorine**, **cobalt**, **tin** and **zinc** are found in many foods: These minerals are essential but are rarely lacking in the human diet.

Water is the last important nutrient mentioned in this section, but it's by no means the least important. Your body is made up of 60 per cent or more water and all the nutrients in your body are dissolved in it. You need to drink about six to eight glasses, or one and a half to two litres, of fluid per day — more if the weather is very hot or you're exercising a lot.

You can live without food for some time, but you'll not last long without water. Water can help to give a feeling of fullness that reduces appetite.

Considering the effect of alcohol

Alcohol is high in kilojoules but offers no particular nutritional value, although it has been shown that a moderate amount (a small glass or two of wine a day) may reduce the risk of heart attack. Unfortunately, alcohol is often taken to excess and does major damage to the body; it can damage the liver, brain and pancreas (where insulin comes from!).

Because alcohol has kilojoules, if you drink some, you must consider it as extra kilojoules in your diet. Replacing food kilojoules with alcohol kilojoules may mean your diet becomes inadequate in valuable vitamins and minerals. If you drink alcohol, limit your intake to no more than two standard drinks five out of seven days per week. In Australia, a standard drink is the volume of an alcoholic beverage which provides 10 grams of alcohol.

The kilojoule content of one standard drink from the more common alcoholic beverages is

- 30 millilitres of most spirits contain 252 kilojoules
- 60 millilitres of dry sherry contain 252 kilojoules
- 100 millilitres of red or white wine contain 285 kilojoules
- 60 millilitres of port or sweet sherry contain 378 kilojoules
- 285 millilitres of full-strength beer contain 491 kilojoules
- 425 millilitres of low-alcohol beer contain 438 kilojoules

In addition to the kilojoules, alcohol plays other roles in diabetes. If alcohol is taken without food, it can cause low blood glucose by increasing the effect of insulin without food to compensate. Hypoglycaemia after drinking alcohol can occur in people with type 1 diabetes quite easily. In those with type 2 diabetes, hypoglycaemia after drinking alcohol is less common and usually would only occur in someone taking sulphonylureas or insulin to control blood glucose levels (refer to Chapter 10 for more on medications).

If you're having a couple of glasses of wine or other alcohol, make sure that you eat some carbohydrate-containing food with it, such as crackers or a full meal.

Chapter 12

Keeping It Moving: Exercise Plan

. . . .

In This Chapter

▶ Understanding the importance of exercise

▶ Starting an exercise program — and sticking with it

▶ Burning off that excess weight

▶ Increasing exercise if you have type 1 diabetes

▶ Getting fit if you have type 2 diabetes

▶ Finding the right activity for you

▶ Using weight training to improve your fitness

. . . .

More than 60 years ago, the great leaders in diabetes care declared that proper management has three major aspects:

✔ Proper diet

✔ Appropriate medication

✔ Sufficient exercise

Although exercise was recognised as a key element in the management triad, many people with diabetes remain inactive. We include this chapter in the hope you won't make the same mistake, and cover just how you can incorporate exercise into your daily life, regardless of whether you have type 1 or type 2 diabetes.

Why Exercise Is Important

Regular physical activity has been shown to improve overall health outcomes for people with and without diabetes alike. However, studies have shown that, for people with diabetes, exercise combined with diet and medication improves blood glucose control as well as helps delay macrovascular complications (refer to Chapter 7 for more on these complications).

Getting off the couch: How exercise works its magic

In order to understand how exercise reduces the blood glucose in type 2 diabetes and helps prevent macrovascular disease in both types, you need to have some understanding of the dynamics of metabolism during exercise.

As exercise begins, the demand for both glucose and fat for energy is increased. Glucose and fat leave the sites where they are stored and enter the bloodstream, heading for muscles. At first, glycogen, the storage form of glucose in the liver, begins to break down and release glucose. With continued exercise, glycogen is used up, and the liver begins to make large amounts of glucose from other substances to continue to provide energy.

With steady, ongoing moderate exercise, the glucose production begins to diminish and the body turns to fat for its supply of glucose. This is a wonderful situation, especially if you are trying to lose weight.

On the other hand, if the exercise is very vigorous, the liver actually makes more glucose than the muscles can use immediately, and the blood glucose begins to rise. This explains some of the instances where the glucose is higher after exercise than it is before exercise. The reason the liver makes so much glucose is that very vigorous exercise depletes the stores of glucose in the muscle very rapidly. Vigorous exercise will not be continued for very long, and the extra glucose will be there to replenish the muscle tissue, once exercise ends.

Glucose is a better source of energy when the exercise is very vigorous because it's converted to energy much faster than fat. For less intense exercise, fat is preferred because it provides more energy than an equal amount of glucose.

The feeling of fatigue that occurs with exercise is probably due to the loss of stored muscle glucose. With exercise, insulin levels in people without diabetes and people with type 2 diabetes who don't inject insulin decline because insulin acts to store and not release glucose and fat. Levels of glucagon, adrenaline, cortisol and growth hormone increase to provide more glucose. Studies show that glucagon is responsible for 60 per cent of the glucose, and adrenaline and cortisol are responsible for the other 40 per cent. If insulin did not fall, glucagon couldn't stimulate the liver to make glucose.

You might wonder how insulin can open the cell to the entry of glucose when insulin levels are falling. In fact, three factors are at work here: During exercise, glucose is getting into muscle cells without the need for insulin, the muscle seems to be more sensitive to the insulin, and the rapid circulation that comes with exercise is delivering the smaller amount of insulin more frequently to the muscle. This is exactly what the person with type 2 diabetes hopes to accomplish when insulin resistance is the major block to insulin action. (For more on exercise and type 1 diabetes, see the section 'Exercising if You Have Type 1 Diabetes' later in this chapter.)

Macrovascular disease is prevented in the following ways by exercise, which:

✔ Helps with weight loss in type 2 diabetes

✔ Lowers cholesterol and triglycerides

✔ Lowers blood pressure

✔ Lowers stress levels

✔ Reduces the need for insulin or drugs

Many other studies have shown that exercise helps to normalise blood glucose and reduce haemoglobin A1c in type 2 diabetes. Other benefits include improving muscle strength, increasing bone density and making you feel great!

Getting Started: Exercising When You Have Diabetes

Prior to starting a new exercise program, a person with diabetes who hasn't exercised previously should check with a doctor, especially if over the age of 35 or if diabetes has been present for ten years or longer.

You should check with your GP if you have any of the following risk factors:

✔ A history of coronary artery disease or elevated blood pressure

✔ A physical limitation

✔ Obesity

✔ The presence of any diabetic complications like retinopathy, kidney disease or neuropathy (refer to Chapter 7)

✔ Use of medications

You need to discuss any of these problems with your GP in order to choose the appropriate exercise.

Once exercise is begun, the person with diabetes can do a lot to make it safe and successful. Some important steps to take include

✔ Carrying treatment for hypoglycaemia (if required)

✔ Choosing cotton socks that sit loosely around your legs or ankles, and comfortable, well-fitting shoes suitable for the type of activity

- ✔ Drinking plenty of water
- ✔ Exercising with a friend who knows the signs of hypoglycaemia and how to treat it
- ✔ Not exercising if your blood glucose is greater than 15 mmol/L or if you are feeling unwell
- ✔ Testing the blood glucose more often to understand what happens when you exercise
- ✔ Thinking about the timing, intensity and duration of the exercise
- ✔ Understanding insulin action (if on insulin) and when it is working at its peak
- ✔ Wearing a medical alert bracelet

If you have diabetes, when exercising, you don't need to:

- ✔ Buy special clothing other than the right shoes and socks (and possibly cycle shorts if you are bike riding).
- ✔ Expect to lose certain 'spots' by repetitively exercising them.
- ✔ Exercise to the point of pain.
- ✔ Use exercise gadgets like belts or other objects that don't require you to move.

Getting Your Heart Pumping

To make the most of your exercise, it's important to get your heart pumping at a faster rate, and keep it at that faster rate for a sustained period. Just walking sedately around a shopping centre is not going to make things happen!

Aerobic exercise is exercise that requires oxygen and can be sustained for more than a few minutes, uses major groups of muscles and gets your heart to pump faster during the exercise. We give you many examples of aerobic exercise throughout this chapter. *Anaerobic exercise*, on the other hand, doesn't use oxygen and is brief (sometimes a few seconds) and intense, and usually can't be sustained. Lifting weights or a 100-metre sprint are examples of anaerobic exercise.

To get the most from the activity that you do and start to burn fat, you should try to do exercise that is aerobically based and requires some effort.

The number of kilojoules you use for any exercise is determined by your weight, the intensity of the activity and the time you spend doing it. In order to have a positive effect on your heart, you need to do a moderate level of exercise for 30 to 45 minutes at least three times per week.

Moderate exercise is a moving definition. If you're out of shape, moderate exercise may be slow walking. If you're in good shape, moderate exercise may be jogging or hiking. Moderate exercise is simply something you can do and not get out of breath.

You want to exercise to a level of 'somewhat hard' — about to the point where you're breathing more heavily but can still talk. As you get into shape, the amount of exertion that corresponds to 'somewhat hard' will increase, meaning you need to increase the intensity or duration of your exercise to keep getting the benefits of the exercise.

The choices of activities are really limitless (see the section 'Is Golf a Sport? Choosing Your Activity' later in this chapter for more on this).

Although you only need to do aerobic exercise three or four times per week to have an effect on your heart fitness, a daily program of aerobic exercise has a major impact on your diabetes. Undertaking moderate aerobic exercise for 30 to 45 minutes every day provides enormous physical, mental and emotional benefits.

You should exercise whenever you will do it faithfully. If you like to sleep late but schedule your exercise for 5.30 am, you probably won't consistently exercise, so pick a time that works in with your energy levels. Also bear in mind your eating habits. Your best time to exercise is probably about 60 to 90 minutes after eating because this is when the glucose is peaking, providing the kilojoules you need. Exercising around this period means you avoid the usual post-eating high in your blood glucose and burn up those food kilojoules. You also need to warm up and cool down for about five minutes before and after you exercise.

Even if on holidays, try to keep your regular activity going! It takes only about two to three weeks to lose some of the fitness your exercise has provided. Then it takes up to six weeks to get back to your current level, assuming that your holiday from exercise doesn't go on too long.

Exercising if You Have Type 1 Diabetes

Exercising with type 1 diabetes can be frustrating and complicated, but with careful planning, regular glucose monitoring and helpful advice from your diabetes care team (and sometimes a little bit of trial and error) your exercise can provide you with a whole range of health benefits.

In people without diabetes, insulin secretion is markedly reduced during activity. However, people with type 1 diabetes depend on insulin injections to manage the blood glucose — they don't have the luxury of a 'thermostat' that automatically shuts off during exercise and turns back on when exercise is finished. Once an injection is given, it's active until it is used up.

If you have type 1 diabetes, you need to avoid overdosing on insulin before exercise, which can lead to hypoglycaemia, or underdosing, which can lead to hyperglycaemia.

One recent study showed an 80 per cent reduction of a person's insulin dose allowed the person with diabetes to exercise for three hours, while a 50 per cent reduction forced the person to stop after 90 minutes due to hypoglycaemia. However, each person with type 1 diabetes is different, meaning how your body responds to insulin and exercise is different. The amount you need to reduce your insulin by when exercising will be determined by your individual needs.

You can measure your blood glucose levels before, during and after exercise to help you and your diabetes care team work out how your insulin should be adjusted when you exercise. Once you understand your own blood glucose exercise 'pattern', you can work out your insulin and food strategy.

You may find that different types of activity, and their intensity, have different effects on your blood glucose levels. Exercise of a higher intensity and/or longer duration will mean more glucose used, while sprint activities can increase blood glucose levels initially but they may fall later. Again, once you understand how different activities affect you, you can adjust your insulin accordingly.

Studies have shown that the abdomen is the best site for insulin injection, as this site allows for the most consistent rate of absorption. If you inject into arms or legs prior to exercise, the insulin will be absorbed differently, so only inject into your abdomen when following an exercising regime.

Another way to prevent hypoglycaemia when exercising is to eat or drink some extra carbohydrate. This may be most useful when the exercise is unplanned. You should have a carbohydrate option (one that quickly raises blood glucose) available during or after you exercise. Again, the duration and intensity will determine how much to have.

Hypoglycaemia can occur well after exercise — even the next morning. This is known as *delayed hypoglycaemia*. Keep track of your blood glucose levels after exercising, and have some fast-acting carbohydrates on hand in case your levels start falling. If you do experience delayed hypoglycaemia, adjust your insulin accordingly before undertaking the same sort of exercise next time.

If you have type 1 diabetes, you must test your blood glucose levels before you do any sort of exercise, even if following your usual insulin and food strategy. If your levels are above 15 mmol/L, you should also check your ketone levels. If ketones are present, you shouldn't go ahead with the exercise — the ketones must be cleared first. (Refer to Chapter 9 for more on testing methods.)

Enjoying exercise with type 1 diabetes is a challenge, but a worthwhile one. It requires lots of thought, a degree of planning and practice, practice, practice to get it right! As always, you don't have to do it alone — your diabetes care team are there to help you.

Check out some of the websites listed in Chapter 24 for more advice on and encouragement about exercising when you have type 1 diabetes.

Exercising if You Have Type 2 Diabetes

With sufficient exercise and diet, some people with type 2 diabetes can revert to a non-diabetic state. This doesn't mean that they no longer have diabetes, but it certainly means that they might not develop the long-term complications that can make life so miserable later in life (refer to Chapter 7).

If you haven't already done so, read the sections 'Getting Started: Exercising When You Have Diabetes' and 'Getting Your Heart Pumping' earlier in this chapter for tips on incorporating exercise into your life, and information on the kind of exercise you should be adopting.

Do not continue exercising if you have tightness in your chest, chest pain, severe shortness of breath or dizziness. If you experience any of these symptoms, immediately see your GP or go to the emergency department of your local hospital.

Is Golf a Sport? Choosing Your Activity

While all physical activity is beneficial, you should choose an activity that best meets your goals and is safe for you. The following factors can help you to determine your choice of activity:

✔ Do you like to exercise alone or with company? Pick a competitive or team sport if you prefer company.

✔ Do you like to compete against others or just yourself? Running or walking are sports you can do alone.

✔ Do you prefer vigorous or less vigorous activity? Less vigorous activity over a longer period is just as effective as more vigorous activity undertaken for shorter periods.

✔ Do you live where you can do activities outside all year, or do you need to be inside a lot of the year? Find a sports club, gym or fitness centre if weather prevents year-round outdoor activity.

✔ Do you need special equipment or just a pair of running shoes? Special equipment is very helpful when it's needed.

✔ What benefits are you looking for in your exercise: Cardiovascular, strength, endurance, flexibility or body fat control? You should probably look for all these benefits, but you may have to combine activities to get them all in.

Perhaps a good starting point in your activity selection is to focus on the benefits. Table 12-1 gives you some ideas.

You can tell from Table 12-1 that living in a rural setting where you have plenty of interesting scenery and terrain is helpful because hiking and walking are in practically every list. On the other hand, walking your local streets can be just as enjoyable (and social) and many urban areas now have walking and cycling tracks. You can also use the walking and cycling machines in your local gym, so you don't have to give up exercise if you live in the city.

Table 12-1	Match Your Activity to the Results You Want
If You Want to ...	*Then Consider ...*
Build up cardiovascular condition	Vigorous basketball or netball, squash, hiking, brisk walking, running, dancing, cycling, boxing, soccer
Strengthen your body	Low-size, high-repetition weight-lifting, gymnastics, rock climbing, hiking, brisk walking, yoga
Build up muscular endurance	Rowing, hiking, brisk walking, vigorous basketball or netball, swimming, cycling, boxing
Increase flexibility	Gymnastics, yoga, tae-kwon-do and kick boxing, soccer, surfing, football, Pilates
Control body fat	Squash, singles tennis, hiking, brisk walking, running, dancing, vigorous basketball or netball, walking, cycling

Picking an activity that suits you over the long term

The special needs of many sports (refer to Table 12-1) may turn you off exercising. The curious thing is that the best exercise that you can sustain for life is right at your feet. A brisk daily walk improves heart function, adds to muscular endurance and helps control body fat.

Of course, the social benefits of exercise are very important. You are together with people who are concerned with health and wellbeing. These people usually share many of your interests — for example, the person who likes to jog often likes to hike and climb and go camping. Many lifetime partnerships begin on one side of a tennis court (and some end there as well).

Cross-training, where you do several different activities throughout the week, is a good idea. Cross-training reduces the boredom that may accompany one thing done day after day. It also permits you to exercise regardless of the weather because you can do some things indoors and some outside.

Everything you do burns kilojoules — even sleeping and watching television. But the more you do, and the longer you do it, the more kilojoules you burn.

See Chapter 13 for more help on increasing your motivation to make, and maintain, lifestyle changes.

Taking your current physical condition into account

Your choice of an activity must take into account your physical condition. Certain activities are not suitable for people with certain conditions, especially some of the long-term complications of diabetes (refer to Chapter 7 for more).

If you have diabetic neuropathy and can't feel your feet, you shouldn't do pounding exercises that may damage your feet without your awareness. You can, however, swim, cycle, row or do armchair exercises where you move your upper body vigorously.

If you have diabetic retinopathy, you shouldn't do exercises that raise your blood pressure (like weight-lifting), cause jerky motions in your eyes (like bouncing on a trampoline), or change the pressure in your eyes significantly (like scuba diving or high mountain climbing). You also shouldn't do exercises that place your eyes below the level of your heart, such as when you touch your toes.

If you have kidney disease, you should avoid exercises that raise your blood pressure for prolonged periods. These exercises are extremely intense activities that you do for a long time, like marathon running.

Some people have pain in their legs after they walk a certain distance. This may be due to diminished blood supply to the legs, meaning the needs of the muscles in the legs aren't met by the inadequate blood supply. Although you need to discuss this problem with your doctor, you don't need to give up walking. Determine the distance you can walk up to the point of pain. Walk about three-quarters of that distance and then stop to give the circulation a chance to catch up. Once you have rested, you can go about the same distance again without pain. By stringing several of these walks together, you can get a good, pain-free workout. You may even find that you are able to increase the distance after a while because this kind of training tends to create new blood vessels.

Short of chest pain at rest, which must be addressed by your doctor, no medical condition should prevent you from doing any sort of exercise at all. If you can't work out an exercise that you can do, get together with an exercise physiologist or your local gym instructor. You will be amazed at how many muscles you can move that you never knew you had.

Lifting Weights and Getting Fit

Weight-lifting is a form of anaerobic exercise (refer to the section 'Getting Your Heart Pumping' earlier in this chapter if you're not sure what this is). It involves the movement of heavy weights, which can only be moved for brief periods of time. It results in significant muscle strengthening and increased endurance.

Because weight-lifting causes a significant rise in blood pressure as it is being done, people with severe diabetic eye disease should not do it.

Strength training, which uses lighter weights, can be a form of aerobic exercise. Because the weights are light, they can be moved for prolonged periods of time. The result is improved cardiovascular fitness along with strengthening of muscles, tendons, ligaments and bones. Strength training is an excellent way to protect and strengthen a joint that's beginning to develop some discomfort.

Older people in nursing homes who were given weights of just a few hundred grams have shown excellent return of strength to what appeared to be atrophied muscles. The benefits for you will be that much greater.

Strength training may be good for the days that you don't do your other aerobic exercise, such as walking or cycling, or you can add it for a few minutes after you finish your activity. Strength training is also good for working on a particular group of muscles that you feel is weak. Very often, this muscle is the back. Strength-training exercises can isolate and strengthen each muscle.

If you do a lot of aerobic exercise that involves the legs, you may want to use upper-body strength training only.

Besides the health benefits, physical activity is fun and boosts your mood. It is hard to feel stressed when you're out walking in your favourite park, by the beach or swimming laps in the pool.

Part IV
Living with Diabetes: Your Mental Health

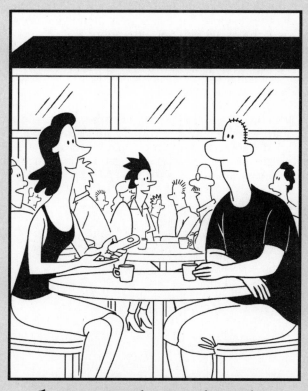

'I stay positive by remembering how sick I was before I was diagnosed.'

In this part ...

Experts now recognise that mental health is a key issue in the management of diabetes and that the less stressed you are, the lower your blood glucose levels and the easier you find it to adopt and maintain required lifestyle changes. However, having diabetes can be emotionally challenging at times. This part provides help with coping with your emotions, as well as methods to keep motivated and positive.

Another objective of this part is to show you that lots of people — some of whom you may not have thought of — are out there to help you manage your diabetes and provide the information that you need to know to assist you in your self-management goals.

Chapter 13

Mint Matters: Mental Health in Diabetes

- -

In This Chapter

▶ Getting to know the mental health problems that commonly occur with diabetes

▶ Understanding how your mental health affects your physical health

▶ Developing coping styles that work over the long term

▶ Incorporating practical coping strategies into your life

▶ Maintaining your enthusiasm for lifestyle changes

▶ Looking at beneficial psychological therapies for people with diabetes

- -

*T*he demands of diabetes can be emotionally challenging at times. You may experience feelings of frustration, anxiety, being burned out from dealing with it, or even symptoms of depression. However, diabetes doesn't need to get you down or get in the way of an enjoyable and rewarding life. While there are certainly challenges to living with diabetes, learning to cope with your emotions can be an important part of maintaining your quality of life.

Mental health is now recognised as a key issue in the management of diabetes. Caring for your mental health in diabetes can also help your physical health. International guidelines for the treatment of diabetes recommend adopting a 'whole-person approach', which involves assessing psychological wellbeing and offering professional psychological support when needed.

In this chapter, we cover ways you can improve your mental health, incorporating healthy coping styles and ideas from psychological therapies, and keep up your motivation to maintain lifestyle changes.

Common Mental Health Problems in Diabetes

A range of emotional reactions are common in diabetes. These can include

- ✔ Anger at the unfairness of being burdened by the diagnosis
- ✔ Disturbances of eating, particularly bingeing
- ✔ Fear — for example, fear of having hypoglycaemia or fear of needles
- ✔ Feeling 'burned out' from dealing with your diabetes
- ✔ Feeling low or depressed
- ✔ Frustration and irritation at the impact of diabetes on your daily routine
- ✔ Guilt and 'beating yourself up' over any contribution of lifestyle factors if diagnosed with type 2 diabetes
- ✔ Mood changes related to variations in your blood glucose levels — for example, feeling nervous when glucose levels are low and down when blood glucose is high
- ✔ Shame, as a result of the stigma of having type 2 diabetes
- ✔ Stress

Everybody experiences emotional ups and downs, and negative emotions can often be short-lived. The following sections cover more serious emotional problems that can occur when you have diabetes, and that can affect your mental and physical health.

If you are experiencing the emotional problems covered in the following sections and these problems are becoming prolonged or interfering with your life, you should seek professional help from your GP or diabetes care team. Discuss with your GP whether a referral to a mental health professional, such as a psychologist or psychiatrist, would be helpful for you.

Depression and diabetes

Studies have shown a link between diabetes and clinical depression, with depression being twice as common in people diagnosed with diabetes, compared to those without.

Clinical depression lasts for at least two weeks and includes at least five of the following symptoms:

- ✔ Changes in appetite, and losing or gaining a significant amount of weight
- ✔ Feeling agitated or sluggish
- ✔ Feeling sad, depressed, empty, anxious or irritable for most of the day, nearly every day
- ✔ Feeling tired and lacking energy
- ✔ Feeling worthless or guilty
- ✔ Having difficulty concentrating or making decisions
- ✔ Having trouble sleeping, or sleeping more than usual
- ✔ Not taking interest in, or getting pleasure out of, daily activities
- ✔ Persistent, negative and repetitive thoughts

Indeed, a two-way relationship has been identified between diabetes and depression: Having diabetes increases the risk of developing depression and having depression increases the risk of developing diabetes. Several possible explanations exist for this connection. For example, feeling low can discourage people from exercising and eating healthily, which can increase the risk of developing diabetes. Or, on the other side of the equation, low blood sugar can cause a dip in mood.

You should not accept depression as 'normal' if you have diabetes. Depression is treatable. Be aware of the symptoms of clinical depression (outlined in the preceding list) and speak to your doctor or diabetes care team if you think that you may be experiencing these symptoms.

Seek professional help immediately from your GP or diabetes care team if you have experienced any thoughts of suicide.

Stress and diabetes

Like depression (see preceding section) stress is another common reaction that has a two-way relationship with diabetes.

Stress can increase your blood glucose levels (see the section 'Blood glucose levels and mental health' for more on this). On the other hand, living with diabetes can at times understandably contribute to the stress in your life. Some experts refer to this as *diabetes-related distress*, which includes worries about living with diabetes, fear of hypoglycaemia and difficulties coping with the diagnosis of diabetes.

See the section 'Working on Practical Strategies for Healthy Coping' for help on reducing your stress levels. For helpful relaxation exercises, see Appendix B.

Connecting Your Mental Health with Your Physical Health

A direct relationship exists between your emotional wellbeing and your physical wellbeing, particularly when you have diabetes. The following sections cover how your mental health can affect your blood glucose levels and your motivation to make and maintain lifestyle changes — and how managing your mental health can therefore improve your physical health.

Blood glucose levels and mental health

Your blood glucose levels are affected by your emotional state. In particular, stress makes the body release hormones such as cortisol and epinephrine, which then pump glucose into blood from storage sites in the liver so the body has more energy available to meet a challenge — meaning stress leads to raised blood glucose.

People who have higher levels of diabetes-related distress (such as worries about living with diabetes and difficulty coping with the condition and its treatment) also tend to have higher blood glucose levels.

This means addressing stress is not only good for your quality of life, but also has the potential to improve your blood glucose levels. Research has found that people with diabetes who participated in a stress-management program significantly improved their blood glucose levels.

Lifestyle changes and mental health

Depression and anxiety can make it more difficult to carry out self-management of diabetes. Feeling low can make you less motivated to exercise, take medications and take good care of yourself, which can put your physical and mental health at risk, which can then add to your distress. People who are chronically depressed also tend to have higher blood pressure and are more prone to heart disease.

The good news is that this cycle of diabetes and depression can be reversed. By taking steps to use more helpful ways of coping with diabetes (outlined in this chapter) and by treating mental illness, you can improve your mental health, increase your confidence in managing your diabetes and increase your motivation for self-care and lifestyle changes, such as exercise. These changes, in turn, can improve your physical health, which can give a further lift to your mental health.

Adopting Healthy Coping Styles

You can manage stress using a variety of coping styles, both healthy and unhealthy. Adopting a healthy coping style for dealing with stress and other emotional problems in your life is particularly important when you have diabetes.

When looking at the range of coping styles available, *coping* refers to the variety of mental and behavioural strategies individuals can use to manage stress, meaning *coping styles* are the behaviours you can adopt to offset or overcome difficult or stressful situations. Coping styles relate to how you react to a problem — they don't actually eliminate the underlying problem. Some coping styles are more effective and adaptive than others.

Coping styles are often divided into emotion-focused coping and problem-focused coping. Emotion-focused coping incorporates efforts to manage the negative thoughts and feelings associated with the stressor. These can be *adaptive* (such as meditating, using relaxation techniques, walking, asking for support from friends and family) or *maladaptive* (such as picking a fight, drinking too much alcohol, taking up smoking or gambling). Problem-focused solving involves attempts to address the source of stress. In the case of diabetes, this could include seeking information about your condition, creating an action plan, learning problem-solving skills, and talking to people living with diabetes about how it affects them.

A maladaptive coping style common among people with diabetes is avoidance. This can be emotional denial (such as telling yourself 'This isn't real'), mental avoidance (such as watching TV to take your mind off things) or behavioural avoidance (such as choosing to sleep for longer periods rather than deal with it). These styles may provide some short-term relief but have been shown to lead to poorer health and more complications further down the track.

While avoiding dealing with your diabetes is an understandable approach, a far more positive coping style is to get on the front foot and learn to deal with issues as they arise. Studies have demonstrated that effective coping is associated with a greater sense of control and self-esteem, lower stress levels and a decreased risk of depression and anxiety.

To consider what coping styles have worked best for you, particularly in times of stress, you can ask yourself the following:

- ✔ What are the biggest challenges I have dealt with so far in my life?
- ✔ What worked? Why? What did I do to help the situation?
- ✔ What didn't? Why? What did I do to hinder the situation?
- ✔ What can I learn from this? What would I do next time?
- ✔ How well do I know myself? What do I need when stressed?
- ✔ What can I learn from others who have been through similar problems?

Recognising effective coping skills is invaluable in helping you deal with the various stages of adjustment to your condition.

Dealing with diabetes involves a number of tasks at different times — these tasks will vary, depending on the stage of your condition.

The first tasks you might have to work through are diabetes-related and include

- ✔ Dealing with self-monitoring
- ✔ Dealing with treatment and lifestyle changes required by your condition
- ✔ Forming and maintaining relations with the health professionals in your diabetes care team
- ✔ Learning to recognise and deal with changes in blood sugar levels

The later tasks you might encounter as you adapt to life with diabetes include

- ✔ Maintaining a healthy lifestyle and keeping up motivation
- ✔ Maintaining relations with family and friends
- ✔ Preserving emotional balance
- ✔ Preserving self-image

Working on Practical Strategies for Healthy Coping

In the following sections we cover techniques to improve your emotional response to stress, and possible problem-focused strategies.

Emotion-focused strategies

Useful emotion-focused methods for achieving emotional balance and allowing emotional expression include the following:

- **Exercising regularly:** Incorporating some moderate exercise into your daily routine has tremendous benefits for both your mental and physical health.

- **Having a list of sayings or affirmations that you find empowering and helpful:** Most people have certain sayings that help them relax, or feel more confident, more focused or less afraid. Be aware of what yours are, write them down and look at them regularly.

- **Keeping a journal:** *Expressive writing* (writing about emotional issues in a personal journal that only you will read) can help you analyse events and how they arose, and can have tremendous benefits for your sense of purpose and sense of control.

- **Practising mindfulness:** Being *mindful* involves disengaging from mental 'clutter' and paying attention to the present moment. Mindfulness helps you to respond rather than react to situations, improving your decision-making skills and increasing your potential for physical and mental relaxation. (See Appendix B for useful mindfulness exercises. For more detailed help with mindfulness, see *Mindfulness For Dummies* by Shamash Alidina (Wiley Publishing Ltd).)

- **Using music strategically:** Certain types of music can help you deal with anxiety, pain and other stressful situations. To get the most out of this strategy, you need to work out what music helps you when stressed, down or fearful, and prepare music collections for those situations.

Practise the techniques included in the preceding list regularly to enhance wellbeing and so they become your automatic response when faced with stressful or problematic situations.

Problem-focused strategies

Problem-focused strategies for dealing with stress can be broken into two main areas: Goal-setting and problem-solving techniques.

Goal-setting techniques

When faced with a problem, one way to work through it is to set clear, achievable goals over a realistic time frame.

When setting a goal for yourself, the goal should be a SMART one. Answer the following questions to make your goal setting more effective:

- ✔ **S = SPECIFIC:** Can I identify my aim? What is it I want to achieve?

- ✔ **M = MEASURABLE:** How will I know when I have achieved my goal? How much? How many?

- ✔ **A = ACHIEVABLE:** Can I achieve this? What do I need?

- ✔ **R = REALISTIC:** Am I being realistic? What are the likely problems? Do I believe this is possible?

- ✔ **T = TIME-BOUND:** Am I willing and able to work for this? Can I do this in a reasonable time frame?

Write down the goals for yourself, your relationships and your work that you'd like to achieve within one week, one month and a time frame of your choosing. Decide what steps you need to take to reach these goals and any problems that may arise. Review your goals on a weekly basis.

Problem-solving techniques

The need for such lifestyle changes as monitoring blood sugars to optimise blood glucose levels, adhering to prescribed dietary regimes and maintaining an exercise schedule can seem burdensome, especially early on. As in other chronic conditions, the daily demands of adhering to treatment regimes and making lifestyle changes require a repertoire of coping strategies.

A healthy coping strategy can be achieved using a problem-solving approach. Tools that can be used in almost any situation include the following:

1. **Clearly identify the problem.**

   You may currently be facing a number of problems. Choose the problem that is troubling you most to work on first — you can come back to your other problems later. Further elaboration of the problem will help to make it clearer to you.

2. **Brainstorm possible solutions to your problem.**

   Now think of as many solutions to your problem as possible —
   including even what may seem wildly unrealistic at first. To help
   generate more possible solutions, think of how one of your friends or
   family members might deal with this problem.

3. **Weigh up the pros and cons of each solution.**

   List the advantages and disadvantages of each solution, rating the
   importance of each advantage or disadvantage on a scale of 0 (not very
   important) to 10 (extremely important).

4. **Decide on the best solution.**

   Now decide which solution is best, having weighed up the pros and
   cons of each. Note that no solution is perfect, and sometimes multiple
   solutions are most useful.

5. **Put your solution into action.**

   List the specific tasks involved in carrying out the best solution and
   set deadlines for these tasks so you get them done. Consider what
   resources are required, who else can help or support you, what
   uncertainties you need to deal with, and/or what you might need to let
   go of to achieve your goal.

6. **Review the problem-solving attempt.**

   Whether the chosen solution was successful or not, review your
   problem-solving technique. This review helps you be better prepared in
   the future and enables you to decide whether another possible solution
   would help with the current problem.

Keeping Up Your Motivation for Lifestyle Changes

Living well with diabetes requires daily attention and self-care, and making
healthy lifestyle changes for the rest of your life. The better you take care of
yourself, the better your quality of life will be, and the less likely you are to
experience complications from diabetes that can lead to suffering.

However, you might feel mixed emotions about taking an active role in
the management of your diabetes. On the one hand, you might find it
empowering to know that making lifestyle changes can lead to a better
outcome for your diabetes. These healthy lifestyle changes, such as regular
exercise and healthy eating, can also improve your physical and mental
health in other ways, outside of the symptoms and complications caused by
having diabetes. On the other hand, it can be challenging, and sometimes
frustrating, to be dedicated to your diabetes care all of the time.

Everybody with diabetes has ups and downs in their commitment to self-care, so it helps to have tips and strategies on hand to give your motivation a boost when it starts to flag. The following sections provide these tips and strategies, using the example of keeping up the motivation to walk for 30 minutes per day. (Of course, you can use these strategies within any aspect of your self-care for diabetes, such as healthy eating or regular blood glucose monitoring.)

Assessing the benefits of lifestyle changes

The benefits and importance of glucose monitoring and other tests, medications, healthy eating and exercise are outlined in the chapters in Part III. However, when looking to maintain your commitment to these areas, it's useful to think of the specific benefits that are the most important to *you*.

For example, the benefits of exercise that are important to you may include reduction in stress and anxiety, improved sleep and increased energy. (Refer to Chapter 12 for more on the benefits of incorporating exercise into your daily life, and help on how to do so.)

Making a list of the pros and cons of a lifestyle change, such as walking each day for 30 minutes, can help to boost your motivation. In this example, short-terms costs may include having to buy new shoes and feeling uncomfortable, whereas short-term benefits may include feeling refreshed and happier, and long-term benefits may include weight loss and an increase in energy.

Increasing your motivation to change

To build up your enthusiasm for making and maintaining lifestyle changes — and to quickly restore it if it starts to weaken — keep the following in mind:

✔ **Set goals in collaboration with your diabetes care team.** Objectives for your self-care (including blood-glucose targets, healthy eating plan and exercise plan) should be set with your team of diabetes health professionals to ensure that the goals are safe and the plans are the best options for you. Your diabetes care team will also help you set smaller goals within each of your larger goals. Setting smaller goals will help ensure you feel your goals are achievable, which in turn will help you stay motivated.

✔ **Use confidence and importance 'rulers'.** You are most likely to meet a goal if you believe both that the goal is important and that you can meet it. You can rate how important you believe your lifestyle goal to be on to a 'ruler' of numbers between 0 and 10, with 0 being 'not at all important' and 10 being 'very important'.

✔ **Monitor your progress using a daily diary.** To evaluate your progress, keep a daily diary of the changes you've made to achieve the goal you're working towards (for example, an exercise diary that includes your pedometer readings each day). Even just keeping this diary can keep up your motivation.

✔ **Recognise the progress that you've made and give yourself rewards.** Particularly when making challenging changes, be sure to recognise when you've made progress and met your goals, and treat yourself with a healthy reward such as a massage or movie.

✔ **Maintain your objectivity.** You may find that, like most people with diabetes, you are more effective with some parts of your self-care than others. For example, perhaps you forget to take your insulin or medication, but have been keeping up your healthy eating plan. Try to be objective, giving yourself credit for lifestyle changes that you've been doing well at, while also identifying ones that you need to work on more.

✔ **Review the pros and cons.** Look over your lists of short-term and long-term costs and benefits to remember the reasons for changing your lifestyle that are most important to you.

✔ **Identify barriers and find solutions.** Like most people, you can probably identify some barriers to making (or keeping up) your lifestyles changes for diabetes self-care. Write down suggested solutions for each of the barriers you find. It can also be useful to anticipate 'high-risk' situations in which you might find it more difficult to keep up your healthy lifestyle and to plan for these. Ask yourself when you think you would be more likely to let your exercise plan or healthy eating plan slip. Examples of possible situations include when it's raining (making it hard to do your usual exercise) or when you're busy at work or on holidays (making it difficult to keep up healthy eating and regular exercise).

✔ **Seek support from family and friends.** You don't have to do it alone! Talk to family and friends about your exercise or healthy eating program and ask for their support. Ask a friend or family member to join you in your exercise program, to call you and encourage you, or to ask you for updates on your progress. Join a walking group or set one up yourself. Speak to other people with diabetes about their experiences. Ask your diabetes nurse educator or diabetes association for information about support groups for people with diabetes in your area. Even just knowing that somebody else is interested can keep your motivation up.

✔ **Get professional support.** A range of professionals with expertise in assisting people with diabetes are available to help you keep up healthy lifestyles. For example, exercise physiologists can help you develop an exercise plan tailored to your needs — one that's safe, enjoyable and designed to be incorporated easily into your everyday life. Psychologists, counsellors and mental health workers can assist you in building and keeping up motivation for your lifestyle goals, particularly if you find that symptoms of depression or anxiety are getting in the way of making changes.

Maintaining healthy lifestyle changes

Living with diabetes requires keeping up healthy lifestyle changes for life. While it is one thing to adjust to a new lifestyle of dedicated self-care, sometimes maintaining your motivation for self-care over the years can be even harder. The good news is that parts of your healthy lifestyle changes for diabetes care — such as regular exercise — can become habits ingrained in your everyday life.

However, you may find that you gradually become sick and tired, or perhaps frustrated, with keeping up your diabetes self-care. If so, you may be experiencing what some experts refer to as *diabetes burnout*, or loss of motivation for management of diabetes. Diabetes burnout is not depression, but is a temporary fatigue or discouragement with your diabetes.

If you find that your motivation is waning and you're slipping from your exercise plan, healthy eating plan or other parts of your self-care program, take stock and speak to your diabetes care team. You can also keep in mind the following tips:

✔ **Don't beat yourself up.** Remember that almost everybody with diabetes experiences lapses in motivation for self-care. This is understandable. Give yourself some credit for the efforts that you *have* made. Rather than dwelling on feelings of guilt or helplessness, focus on getting support to move forward. Accepting your condition is an important part of moving forward.

✔ **Pretend you're starting over.** Review your list of the benefits of making healthy lifestyle changes for diabetes, and your confidence and importance 'rulers' (see the preceding section).

✔ **Review your goals with your diabetes care team.** Discuss the priorities that you would like to work on first. Remember to tell the significant people in your life about your self-care plans, and ask them to help you to keep them up.

Finding Psychological Therapies That Work with Diabetes

Depression, anxiety and other psychological problems common in people with diabetes are treatable. The treatment of psychological problems and diabetes involves a coordinated approach that monitors both diabetes control and mental health. The most effective treatments combine psychological and medical care.

Psychological support can also assist with adjusting to living with diabetes and making lifestyle changes, such as adopting healthier eating and increasing exercise.

Different types of psychological therapies are available, provided by a range of mental health professionals that includes psychologists, clinical psychologists, counsellors and psychiatrists. Most psychological therapies involve a structured approach to 'talking therapy' and involve learning and practising new skills.

Research has shown two types of psychological therapies are particularly helpful for people with diabetes, especially in specific areas. Motivational interviewing can assist in making lifestyle changes, while cognitive behaviour therapy has been found to be useful for people with diabetes experiencing depression.

If you are experiencing self-blame, persistent, negative and repetitive thoughts, suicidal thoughts, very poor sleep or other signs of significant depression or anxiety (or another psychological disorder), see your GP or a mental health professional for an assessment. (Refer to the section 'Depression and diabetes' earlier in this chapter for a full list of the signs of clinical depression.)

Motivational approaches

Motivational interviewing is a psychological approach that focuses on increasing motivation to change behaviour. This counselling style has been used effectively for a range of different situations that require people to change their behaviour, including alcohol and drug abuse, smoking, weight loss, increasing physical activity and adherence to treatments for medical conditions.

The management of diabetes requires lifelong changes in behaviour, and people vary in how ready they are to make these changes. Motivational interviewing is used to assist people with diabetes in building up and maintaining their motivation and confidence in making these lifestyle changes.

Many self-help strategies are available that help you build your motivation to make the lifestyle changes required for your diabetes management. In particular, you can use these strategies when approaching the areas of diabetes self-care that you sometimes find difficult to keep going with (or to start!). (For information on these self-help strategies, refer to the section 'Increasing your motivation to change' earlier in this chapter.)

Talk with your GP or diabetes care team if you'd like some extra tips on increasing and maintaining your motivation, setting realistic goals, or if you'd like to be referred to a psychologist or counsellor who specialises in motivational interviewing for making lifestyle changes, improving weight management or assisting with chronic disease or health-related problems.

Cognitive behavioural therapy

Cognitive behavioural therapy (CBT) is one of the most widely researched psychological treatments for depression and anxiety. CBT focuses on the interconnected nature of our thoughts (or interpretations), behaviours and feelings (or emotions). Thoughts influence feelings, and vice versa. The way we act (our behaviour) can also reinforce, or change, our thoughts and feelings. Thoughts, feelings and behaviours all play important roles in the development and maintenance of depression and anxiety.

While different forms of this therapy are available for the treatment of specific problems, all forms of CBT use techniques to help you change the way you think, and also gradually change the way you behave, to make you feel better.

The following sections outline some strategies used in CBT for depression. This isn't a comprehensive guide to CBT self-treatment; however, some examples of techniques are provided that you may find useful. For more information on CBT, see *Cognitive Behavioural Therapy For Dummies*, 2nd Edition, by Rhena Branch and Rob Willson (Wiley Publishing Ltd).

Recognising the links between thoughts and feelings

For any event or situation, you have thoughts (or interpretations) about that situation, which in turn lead to your feelings (emotions). Different people will often come to different interpretations of the same situation, meaning situations themselves don't directly lead to specific feelings — although sometimes your thoughts might be so quick that you're barely able to catch them.

For example, imagine that you arrange to meet a friend to go to the movies, but they're running late. What would you be thinking and feeling? One reaction might be sadness (your friend is late because he didn't actually want to come), despair (you knew your friend didn't actually like you; no-one does) or anxiety (your friend has been in an accident). But another reaction could simply be mild annoyance and the assumption that your friend is caught in traffic.

As you can see from this example, one event can be viewed from several different perspectives. Some interpretations lead to distressing feelings, while others don't. It can then become a cycle — a person who is feeling depressed is more likely to interpret situations in a way that leads to further sadness.

However, CBT works to interrupt this cycle by changing unhelpful thoughts that lead to distressing feelings. The first step to challenging any unhelpful or unrealistic thoughts is to catch the thoughts that you're having.

Monitoring your thoughts and feelings

A core element of CBT is increasing your awareness of the links between your thoughts, feelings and events in your life. A good way to do this is to keep a daily record of your thoughts and feelings. While this may seem simple, many people find it difficult to identify their feelings or to distinguish between different feelings.

Catching thoughts, which often occur very quickly, can be even more difficult at first. Thoughts aren't always that obvious. By keeping a record, you can practise clearly identifying your thoughts and feelings.

When writing up your daily record, include the following:

- **Events:** Write down the event that occurred just before you experienced your feeling. Sometimes you may notice your feelings first, so you may need to work backwards and think about what happened before your feeling. In some cases, it may simply be that a thought came into your mind.

- **Feelings:** Write down negative feelings (emotions) you felt that day and rate them on a scale from 1 (very mild) to 100 (very severe). It's common to experience several feelings at once, so make sure you write them all down. Negative feelings include sadness, despair, anger, annoyance, frustration, fear, anxiety, shame, embarrassment, helplessness and hopelessness. Also include some examples of when you felt strong, positive emotions during the day, such as happiness, contentment, excitement, pride or relaxation.

- **Thoughts:** These are the interpretations that you had about the event and can be hard to identify at first. If you're struggling to catch your thought process, ask yourself what somebody else in that situation might have been thinking that would lead to that feeling.

Identifying distorted thoughts in depression

Thoughts often seem like facts, especially when they come very quickly. However, most thoughts are interpretations that don't necessarily match reality. A range of different interpretations are possible for every situation and, when people are feeling depressed, they tend to interpret situations in particular, biased, ways that are more likely to lead to feelings of sadness. These are known as *distorted thoughts*.

The next step in CBT is to examine your thoughts to see if any distorted thoughts are apparent that are leading to distressing feelings.

Picking up on your distorted thoughts allows you to reflect on and weigh up your thoughts to see if they match reality.

Common types of distortions in thinking are:

- **Black-and-white or all-or-nothing thinking:** With this type of thinking, everything is polarised into one extreme or the other, without any shades of grey in between. For example, 'My results will be either perfect or a failure'. This type of thinking can be a problem because it sets people up for a sense of disappointment or failure.

- **Overgeneralising:** With this type of thinking, a single event is interpreted as always being the case and the way that things will always be. For example, one mistake is interpreted as, 'I always do everything wrong', or one occasion of eating unhealthy food is interpreted as, 'I can never stick to my healthy eating plan'.

- **Jumping to conclusions:** With this type of thinking, the mind jumps to the conclusion of a negative thought, without stopping to consider the evidence. For example, 'That was my fault', when evidence to the contrary can be identified.

- **Dismissing the positive evidence:** This type of distorted thinking happens when you see the positive evidence, but your mind doesn't let you believe it. For example, if several people compliment you by telling you that you're hard working, your mind dismisses this by saying, 'Oh, I'm not really hard working; they're just being polite. What they really mean is that I'm not smart so have to try hard to make up for it'.

- **Mind-reading:** This occurs when you assume that you know what another person is thinking. For example, 'She did that because she doesn't like me and was trying to avoid me'.

Everybody has distorted thoughts. The key is to be able to to pick up on them and work out how they're leading to distressing feelings and, ultimately, influencing your behaviour.

Challenging distorted and unhelpful thoughts

Once you have identified any distorted or unhelpful thoughts, the next step is to challenge these thoughts when they arise. The aim is not simply 'positive thinking' or to be unrealistic. Instead, you should aim to have balanced thoughts that match reality as closely as possible.

Once you have identified a thought leading to a negative feeling (such as sadness or anxiety), you can ask yourself:

- ✔ Is there a distortion in this thought?

- ✔ Is there any evidence that contradicts this? If I was in a court of law, what would the other side say to prove that this thought is not true?

- ✔ Do I have any experiences that would contradict this thought in any way?

- ✔ Is there another, more helpful, way of viewing this situation that takes into account more evidence and doesn't lead to negative feelings?

The theories behind CBT are about helping you to know yourself better, particularly to work out how you deal with stress, anxiety and depression. The techniques described are really basic life skills that are useful in a broad range of situations and can be used to help build your confidence in dealing with both your diabetes and other life situations. The trick is to establish what works best for you as an individual.

Talk with your GP or diabetes care team if you'd like a referral to a psychologist or counsellor specialising in CBT for depression or anxiety.

Chapter 14

Diabetes Is Your Show

. . . .

In This Chapter

▶ Presenting you — the author, the producer, the director and the star

▶ Using your GP — your assistant director

▶ Taking advantage of the diabetes specialist or endocrinologist — your technical consultant

▶ Seeing your eye doctor — your lighting designer

▶ Employing your foot doctor — your dance instructor

▶ Engaging your dietitian — your food services director

▶ Getting information from your diabetes educator — your researcher

▶ Listening to the pharmacist — your usher

▶ Using your mental health worker — your supporting actor

▶ Inviting your family and friends — your captivated and caring audience

. . . .

Shakespeare said it: 'All the world's a stage'. Certainly your diabetes fits that description beautifully. You have many roles in life, and one of them is the role of a person with diabetes. (The others may include brother or sister, mother or father, boss or employee, and so on.) As with any role, you're not expected to play your role as a person with diabetes by yourself. You have a large cast and crew, all of whom are eager to help you — as long as you're willing to ask for their help and know how to make use of their talents, they can give you their best. As members of that crew, we know everyone wants to give you his or her best.

In this chapter, we take you through all the cast and crew available to help you make the most of your management of your diabetes.

You Are the Author, the Producer, the Director and the Star

Being the author, the producer, the director and the star may seem like a lot of responsibility — and it is. Unlike many short-term illnesses where the doctor knows what has to be done, instructs you to do it, writes a prescription, and you're cured, diabetes is your daily companion for life. No-one, not even your mother or spouse, can be with you all of the time. Therefore, you're the one who writes the script and the action. You decide whether you'll take your medication or exercise regularly. You determine whether you'll follow a healthy eating plan that will help control your weight and your blood glucose.

You're the one who needs to gather the resources required to play the role properly. In this sense, you're the producer. You need your props and your theatre, the equipment, the medications and the environment in which to manage your diabetes. Your environment may be a comfortable home where you can eat the proper diet and with a good exercise facility where you can burn up kilojoules while you strengthen your heart. Or it may just be the footpath or park where you can safely walk or jog.

Once you have the resources, you need to direct your cast and crew to make your play come out the way you envision it. You're the one who sees to it that your GP obtains a glycosylated HbA1c every three or four months and that he or she sends you to the eye doctor at least once a year. The doctor is dealing with many patients each day and can easily forget your specific needs. You must let the doctor know what your needs are and not expect the doctor to read your mind. You may be dealing with other doctors who treat your heart, your lungs and other parts of you. Each doctor needs to know all the medications you take.

Finally, you're the star of the show. That role is both an honour and a responsibility. Although you may wish that you had never been chosen for this particular role, there it is. You can make of it what you will. You can learn all your lines (understand your disease) and speak them fluently (take your medications, do some exercise, and so on), or not. Obviously, not studying your lines is a lot easier, but in that case, the resulting production may not be up to the standard that you want. Take proper care of yourself, and the smile on your face and that of all your fellow cast members and crew will clearly indicate that you have written, produced, directed and starred in the production of a lifetime.

The General Practitioner — Your Assistant Director

Your GP takes on a new role in diabetes, where he or she becomes a facilitator. In Australia, where you can find numerous specialist doctors, only a small percentage of people with diabetes see a diabetes specialist regularly. The large majority of people with diabetes, especially type 2, are in the hands of their local GPs who have to deal with many other illnesses besides diabetes. This is a consequence of the large size of the population with diabetes and the requirements of the healthcare system.

While using a GP instead of a specialist may not seem conducive to the best care, it has many benefits. Remember, you're a person who has diabetes. Other things can go wrong, and your GP can handle them as well. Your mild heart disease may not require a cardiologist and can be handled by your GP; your GP can also manage your bronchitis very well.

GPs can provide you with access to Medicare-funded visits to dietitians, diabetes educators, podiatrists and psychologists. In some cases, the Medicare refund doesn't cover the entire cost of these visits and you have to pay the difference. Alternatively, your GP can refer you to a diabetes centre or service at the local health centre or attached to your local hospital. These visits are free.

You should expect your GP to have a decent working knowledge of diabetes and know the proper way to treat a person with diabetes. Various tests are essential to monitor your health, and your GP must know which ones to order and when to send you to a specialist in situations where your needs are beyond your GP's expertise. For example, your GP should be aware of the necessity to regularly take tests for early warning signs of kidney damage (refer to Chapter 7).

The Diabetes Specialist or Endocrinologist — Your Technical Consultant

Your diabetes specialist or endocrinologist should have the most in-depth knowledge of the management of diabetes. This medical care person has had advanced training for several years after the years of training in general internal medicine and has devoted years to taking care of people with diabetes plus a few other kinds of patients. The *diabetes specialist* is an endocrinologist who only takes care of patients with diabetes, and not thyroid cases or adrenal cases or diseases of other glands of the body.

The person with type 1 diabetes will certainly see an endocrinologist sooner or later. If the person with type 2 diabetes gets into trouble with complications or control, the endocrinologist will be called in for consultation. You have the right to expect that this doctor will be able to answer most questions that arise during the care of diabetes.

The diabetes specialist will be conversant with the newest treatments for diabetes, so if you have questions about the future of diabetes care, ask them. This doctor should also have the best understanding of all the drugs currently used for diabetes, how they interact with each other, their side effects and other drugs that interact with them.

If you're not satisfied with the answers you're getting from your GP, ask your GP for a referral to a specialist. Make sure that any changes in your treatment or medication that the endocrinologist makes are reported to your GP. One of the big problems in medicine is the lack of communication between medical care providers of all types, not just doctors.

For your own sake, make sure that all your medical care providers know what the others are doing for you.

The Eye Doctor — Your Lighting Designer

The eye doctor (*ophthalmologist*) is the one who ensures that your diabetes will not damage your vision. This doctor is a medical specialist who has received advanced training in diseases of the eye. Your general practitioner must see (no pun intended) to it that you have an examination by this specialist at least once a year and more often if necessary.

An ophthalmologist must usually dilate the pupils of the eyes with drops in order to do a proper examination.

The ophthalmologist examines you for the conditions we outline in Chapter 7. The ophthalmologist must send a report to your GP and should also take the opportunity to educate you about diabetic eye disease.

Sometimes the good deed of restoring vision leads to unexpected consequences. It's not uncommon for the ophthalmologist to repair your cataracts, only to find that behind all that fuzz was diabetic retinopathy — which then itself needs to be assessed and treated.

In Australia, screening for diabetic eye disease can now also be performed by well-trained optometrists, who may use a retinal camera without eye drops. If the optometrist detects anything concerning, you will be referred to a specialist ophthalmologist. Seeing an optometrist is Medicare-funded and most optometrists bulk bill.

The Foot Doctor — Your Dance Instructor

The foot doctor or podiatrist is your best source of help with the minor and some of the major foot problems that all people suffer. You should go to a podiatrist with such problems as toenails that are hard to cut, corns and calluses, and certainly any ulcer or infection of your foot. This is especially true if you have any neuropathy (refer to Chapter 7). In that case, you're better off not trying to cut your toenails by yourself.

Podiatrists we speak with emphasise that the earlier a potential problem is properly attended to, the less likely it is that a minor problem turns into a major disaster.

The podiatrist can tell you which preparations you should not use on your skin and can show you how important it is that you give lesions time to heal and not to rush to put weight on your injured feet. Many podiatrists also give you a list of dos and don'ts for the proper care of your feet, such as examining feet daily, avoiding extreme heat, and so on. Chapter 8 details all the things you need to do to preserve good foot health.

The Dietitian — Your Food Services Director

This person undertakes one of the most important roles in your care. Because most people with diabetes have type 2 and type 2 is greatly worsened by being overweight, a good dietitian can really help you to control your blood glucose both by eating the right foods and amounts and helping you to lose weight. The dietitian can also show you which foods belong to which energy source — carbohydrate, protein and fat — and generally ensure your diet is totally adequate for your individual needs. (Refer to Chapter 11 for more on your diet.)

The person with type 1 diabetes needs to know how food interacts with insulin injections. The dietitian can teach you to count carbohydrates so that you know how much insulin to take for your meals. (Refer to Chapter 11 for more information.)

Most ethnic foods can be incorporated into a healthy eating plan, even if the recipe needs a little tweaking. This means that you can still enjoy the foods you have always eaten while you stay within the bounds of a healthy diet. A good dietitian is the best source for this kind of information.

One thing you want to be sure of is that the dietitian has a flexible approach to food. The dietary information you are ultimately given should take into account your preferences as well as the fact that the right amount of carbohydrate, protein and fat is different for different individuals. Any dietitian who simply hands you a printed diet and says, 'Follow this' is doing you no favours.

Diabetes Centres will have specialist diabetes dietitians available. You can also find private-practice dietitians who specialise in diabetes on the DAA or ADEA websites (see Chapter 24). Seeing an accredited practising dietitian (APD) is your guarantee of quality, as these dietitians undertake regular professional development and training.

The Diabetes Educator — Your Researcher

Every person in your play is actually an educator in addition to their other role, but diabetes educators are specially trained to teach you what you need to know about every aspect of diabetes so that you properly take care of yourself. They should have CDE (Credentialled Diabetes Educator) after their names. A CDE has taken an extensive course in diabetes and undertakes regular professional development to remain up to date in diabetes management. A diabetes educator teaches you how to take your insulin or tablets, how to test your blood glucose and how to acquire any of the other skills you need.

You can find many diabetes educators in a Diabetes Education Centre. Once you have got over the shock of having diabetes, asking your GP to refer you to such a centre is a good idea. After you have visited the centre, go back regularly and update yourself. New drugs and new procedures are constantly being discovered. The diabetes educator can be a wonderful source of information about these, while making sure that you continue in your good habits. The Australian Diabetes Council in NSW or Diabetes Australia in your state or territory can assist you to find a Diabetes Education Centre close to you.

The Pharmacist — Your Usher

The role of the usher may not sound important, but how will you enjoy the play if you can't find your seat? The pharmacist is your guide to all the medications and tools required to control your blood glucose and manage any complications that you develop, ushering you into the use of all these strange and new products. You may see your pharmacist more often than you see other members of your cast and crew in the medical field.

Each time you start a new medication, a good pharmacist checks to make sure that it doesn't conflict with other medicines you are taking. The pharmacist tells you about side effects and makes sure that your doctor is checking you for adverse drug reactions or interactions. The pharmacist may give you a printout that you can take home and refer to, telling you all you need to know about your new medication.

Many pharmacists also prepare a list of medications that you take, telling you each drug's strengths and dosage frequency. You can carry this around in case anyone ever needs to know what you take.

Pharmacists can tell you about helpful over-the-counter drugs that are available without prescription. A pharmacist can also visit you at home to help you get the best from your medication; this service is called a *home medicines review* and can be organised free of charge with your local doctor.

The Mental Health Worker — Your Supporting Actor

Your mental health worker may be a psychiatrist, a psychologist, a counsellor or a social worker — or your GP may play this role. This person comes in handy whenever you have times when you feel you just can't cope. (Refer to Chapter 13 for more about dealing with the emotional aspects of diabetes.) The mental health worker is there at those times to support you and get you going again. Diabetes certainly proves the theory that all disease is both physical and emotional.

Your Family and Friends — Your Captivated and Caring Audience

Your audience is the people you live with, work with and play with. Your family and friends can be a tremendous source of help, so let them know that you have diabetes. If you have type 1 diabetes, you can teach them how to recognise when your glucose is too low, in case you're ever too ill to take care of yourself. If you're type 2, ask your family to moderate their diet to help you follow yours. The healthy eating guidelines for people with diabetes are good for everyone. Complying with your diet can be difficult enough, without your family enjoying high-kilojoule foods in front of you!

Your family or friends can also become your exercise partners. Sticking to a program is a lot easier when a partner is counting on you to show up to work out. Your family and friends can also accompany you when you visit the doctor and remind you to ask the doctor a question or to follow the instructions you received.

Let these people know about your diabetes and give them a copy of this book so that they understand something about what you're going through and how they can best help you.

Chapter 15

Putting Your Knowledge to Work for You

*I*f you read Parts III and IV of this book, you will know as much as the experts. But knowing is often quite a different thing to doing. If this were not the case, the world would be a much better place to live in because in most cases everyone would know what they needed to do, even if they didn't do it.

The key thing is to get going on your required lifestyle changes now. Don't wait another day to begin to do the things that can prolong your life and increase its quality at the same time. This chapter shows you how.

Developing Positive Thinking

Studies have shown fairly conclusively that if you start with a positive frame of mind, your body can work with you and not against you. Even when things go wrong, if you're optimistic, you can pick yourself up and move forward. If you're pessimistic, you can become depressed and believe that nothing will help you. That kind of attitude is not conducive to good control of your blood glucose and avoidance of complications.

Maintaining a positive attitude has a lot to do with how you interpret problems. If you view problems as permanent and unchangeable, then you will have trouble being positive. If you view problems as temporary setbacks that can be overcome, given enough time, you will be much more optimistic and able to enjoy life more.

Positive thinking doesn't come naturally to everyone. If you're struggling with negative feelings and emotions about your diabetes, please seek help from the many health care professionals available to provide support (refer to Chapter 13 for self-help strategies and more on the support options available).

Monitoring and Testing

Many of our patients ask us about a cure for diabetes. One doesn't exist yet, but the future looks very promising. So far, doctors don't have a portable machine that can measure the blood glucose and respond with the right amount of insulin (this would be an artificial pancreas and we don't have these yet!). Therefore, you and your diabetes care team have to make the calculations that your pancreas would do automatically if it could. The calculations are, of course, how much medicine to take for a given glucose. To make these calculations, you and the team need to know the blood glucose levels. This is where monitoring comes in.

If you have type 1 diabetes, you should monitor before meals and at bedtime at least. If you have type 2 diabetes, you can get away with a single daily test — unless you're on insulin, in which case an extra reading or two each day is a good idea. Chapter 9 is where you can find what you, with the help of your GP or diabetes care team, should do in response to your glucose test results. What you look for are trends in your blood glucose readings, and your GP, diabetes educator and/or dietitian can help you to see and analyse trends.

Blood glucose tests are only a moment in time, however. What you need to know is whether you have good control 24 hours a day. That is where the glycosylated HbA1c comes in (refer to Chapter 9). Your doctor should order this test every three to four months if you're stable and every three months if not. If you have close to normal results in this test, you can reduce your worry about long-term complications (refer to Chapter 7) and will probably not be experiencing short-term complications, either (refer to Chapter 6).

Even with near-normal glycosylated HbA1c results, you still want to be checked for any sign of complications. That means regular eye examinations, regular blood and urine tests for kidney damage, and regular tests for sensation in your feet (refer to Chapter 14). Your doctor should do this on schedule; if not, you have to remind the doctor.

Effective treatment exists for the majority of the complications of diabetes, and the earlier the treatment is started, the less likely it is that the complication will lead to serious damage. Routine monitoring and testing allow you to discover the problem as early as possible.

Table 15-1 provides a comprehensive checklist of all the tests you should be having and how often.

Table 15-1	Responsibilities and Required Tests When Diagnosed with Diabetes

Your responsibilities when diagnosed with diabetes

Keep a logbook or diary on a daily basis of your blood glucose results.

Maintain a healthy diet and the best body weight that you can.

Participate in regular physical activity.

Wash and inspect your feet daily.

Maintain, store and take your medications correctly.

Wear a medical alert bracelet and carry hypoglycaemia treatment (such as sweets and other food) with you if you are on insulin or oral hypoglycaemic tablets.

Notify the motor vehicle licensing department and your insurance company.

Register with the National Diabetes Services Scheme.

Monitor your blood glucose regularly.

Have your eyes checked every year.

Visit your doctor before you become pregnant to work out a plan to keep you and the baby healthy.

Visit your doctor and other members of your health team regularly.

Your doctor's responsibilities when you have a diagnosis of diabetes

Perhaps keep a diabetes register to keep track of patients with diabetes, including a recall system to send out reminders for visits.

Keep well-organised patient records to allow easy tracking of blood glucose results over time.

(continued)

Table 15-1 *(continued)*

Your doctor's responsibilities at your three- to four-monthly review

Assess blood glucose results direct from meter or your logbook.

Review medications and frequency of blood glucose monitoring.

Check any new medications for possible interactions with diabetes treatment.

Assess diet (such as fat, fibre and daily carbohydrate intake) and lifestyle choices (such as smoking and consumption of alcohol).

Test for random blood glucose, glycosylated HbA1c or fructosamine.

Record weight/height ratio and blood pressure.

Examine feet and check for wounds, circulation and sensation.

Check injection sites if using insulin.

Check for related illnesses, such as urinary tract infections, or new problems that may interfere with treatment.

Organise referrals to podiatrist, diabetes educator or dietitian, if required.

Your doctor's responsibilities at your annual review

Organise referral to ophthalmologist for full eye exam.

Do a fasting lipid blood test.

Check feet sensation.

Conduct a full cardiovascular assessment — check all pulses and heart.

Conduct a full peripheral nervous system assessment — check sensation and reflexes.

Conduct a full autonomic nervous system assessment — question you about bladder control, sexual function and gut function.

Conduct a full renal assessment.

Using Medications Correctly

Medications can be tricky. Some of them are very potent, but none of them work if you don't take them. Some of the things you need to know when you take your medications include

- Are you taking the right dose at the right time?
- Are you meant to take it with or without food, depending upon the medication?
- Does it mix with your other medications?
- Are you aware of side effects, and are they being monitored?

> ✔ Can the desired effect sometimes be too strong?
>
> ✔ Do you have a readily available antidote to its effect, if necessary?
>
> ✔ Do you need to adjust the dose when you're not feeling well?

Your doctor, your pharmacist and your diabetes educator can all help you with your medications, but you're on your own when it comes to taking them. If you have trouble remembering, get yourself a plastic case containing seven sections with a day of the week written above each section and fill each section with that day's tablets. You can then easily see whether you took them or not. Your pharmacist can also make up these kinds of packs — sometimes called a *blister pack* or *dosette box* — for you. There may be a small charge for this service unless the arrangement is set up using your local doctor.

For more on medications, refer to Chapter 10.

Following a Diet Successfully

Although the emphasis in the last few years has been on reducing fat in your diets, especially cholesterol and saturated fat, when it comes to diabetes, you have to be aware of your carbohydrate intake as well. And it doesn't hurt to know something about the quality of the carbohydrate as well as the quantity. Try to choose low glycaemic index (GI) carbohydrate options — for example, basmati rice instead of white rice. Most carbohydrates with lots of fibre will be a low glycaemic source. You are likely to have a lower blood glucose as a result and may require less insulin to control it. Not only does that mean better control over your diabetes, but your blood fats, particularly triglyceride, are also lower. (Refer to Chapter 11 for more on diet options, including more on low-GI foods.)

Most people can make changes in their diet over the short term, but maintaining these changes over the long term is difficult. The best way to accomplish a long-term change is to have a plan and try to stick to it.

Continue to be 'mindful' of what you are eating over the long term — in other words, regularly pay attention to and reflect on what you're eating to make sure the plan and the reality continue to match up.

It's often the times when you're in an unplanned situation that are the most damaging to your control over diabetes. For example, when you enter a restaurant, you're presented with a menu. The job of the chef is to entice you to order a dish using the description of the food in the menu, just as the pictures on the food packaging in shops are intended to entice you to buy that food. If you have in mind what works in with your healthy eating plan, you tend to order what helps you, not what spoils your control.

An occasional treat can often cheer you up and make the day-to-day job of choosing the best foods more bearable! Your dietitian can help you learn how to manage potentially difficult situations.

Sticking to your eating plan is also important when you eat at someone else's home. Try to select with care, and don't be afraid to say no — try practising it before you leave home! Your dietitian can give you a lot of help about what to select and what to have in small servings or avoid.

One thing that helps a lot in diabetes is having some order in your life. If your life is one of disorganisation, then controlling your diabetes will probably be much more difficult. Your blood glucose control is likely to be better if you take your medications at about the same time each day. Those with type 1 diabetes often manage exercise more easily if it's done at about the same time of the day and on a regular basis. If you have type 2 diabetes and are on oral medications, you may also find it beneficial to eat at a similar time each day. But you don't have to eat the same thing all the time. An endless variety of delicious foods is available to you — let your dietitian show you the options best for you.

For more on your diet, refer to Chapter 11.

Following an Exercise Program

The more you exercise regularly, the better you can control your blood glucose. This holds true for your weight as well. If you have type 2 diabetes, you need less or no medication. If you have type 1 diabetes, you will need less insulin on the days when you exercise. Your exercise choices are unlimited (refer to Chapter 12).

If you're having trouble exercising, follow these tips:

✔ **Try to do something daily, if possible, or at least three or four times a week.** If you can't exercise regularly on your own, try getting an exercise buddy. You don't need a gym to find step aerobics. Just walk up a few flights of stairs where you work. If the weather permits, go for a walk outside for at least 20 minutes.

✔ **Set up a program with progressive goals so you don't stay stuck at a low level of exercise.** If you don't know how to do this yourself, check with an exercise physiologist. If you're older than 35 and have not exercised and are overweight, check with your doctor before beginning a strenuous program.

✔ **Don't limit yourself to aerobic exercise.** A little strength training or weight-lifting a few days a week can make an amazing difference in your strength, your stamina and your physique. If your sport is tennis, you may find that you can play that third set with much greater ease once you start on a strength-training program. All other sports benefit from strength training in a similar fashion.

Exercise is definitely a way to get high without drugs. It's good for depression or any unhappy state of mind. Don't take our word for it. Get out and find out for yourself. Refer to Chapter 12 for more on exercise.

Using the Expertise of Others

People are usually eager to help you with your diabetes. (Refer to Chapter 14 to find out more about your supporting cast.) So much knowledge is out there, just waiting to be tapped. Medicare and insurance companies recognise the value of resources like a dietitian and are willing to pay for them.

You can get lots of free information from your pharmacist, the internet and other people with diabetes. You may want to be careful of these last two groups, however. A lot of misinformation is shared on the internet and among people with diabetes. Before you make a major alteration in your treatment on the basis of uncertain information, check with your GP or diabetes care team. (You can find out about some of the most common bits of misinformation in Chapters 21 and 23.)

Every time you have a question about your diabetes, write it down and save it for your next visit to your GP or any other diabetes care team member, unless it's urgent. If you don't know whether something is urgent, call your GP or diabetes care team and let them help you to determine the urgency of your problem.

Don't neglect your family and friends as a helpful resource. These are the people who love you and know that you would help them if the tables were turned. The problem is that they can't help you if they don't know what you're dealing with. Tell them that you have diabetes and about the problems, such as hypoglycaemia, that you may face. Tell them how to help you if the need arises. You will find that the result will be a much closer relationship.

Part V
Special Considerations for Living with Diabetes

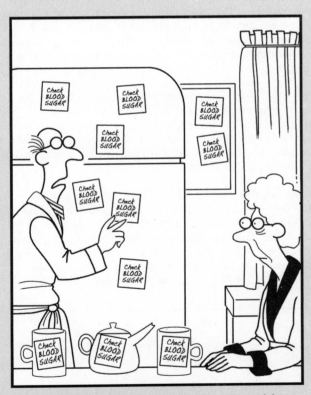

'Do you think the government could include sticky notes in the Pharmaceutical Benefits Scheme?'

In this part ...

Diabetes in growing children and older people often produces problems that the average child or adult doesn't have to deal with. Both groups have emotional problems that are unique. The child is learning to fit in with peers while becoming independent of their parents. Older people may be finishing their working life, downsizing their home and, as they get older, perhaps losing friends and relatives at the same time that their mental processes are declining. This part explains their special problems and how to tackle them.

Another stage of many people's lives is the decision to have children. This part includes a chapter on planning for and dealing with a pregnancy in someone with pre-existing diabetes, helpful to those contemplating this step. Because diabetes can also be diagnosed during pregnancy, we include information on this as well.

Even the middle-aged adult has unique problems, in this case relating to insurance, both life and health, and employment. Fortunately, the barriers are rapidly coming down, but you still need to know about certain issues. Discrimination cannot be tolerated, and you can find out what to do about it here.

Finally, we tell you about the huge number of new developments in medicine, putting them into perspective as to usefulness and appropriateness. After that, we expose the false promises. So many things have been proposed for diabetes care without benefit of careful evaluation. The scientific evidence for and against is presented so that you can make up your own mind.

Chapter 16

Your Child Has Diabetes

. . . .

. . . .

*C*hildren with diabetes present with special issues that adults with diabetes don't have. Not only are they growing and developing from babies to adults, but the problems of psychological and social adjustment can be much harder to handle. Diabetes can cause additional stress at a period of time that's not exactly smooth, even without it.

Members of your diabetes care team understand that if a child has diabetes, the whole family takes on the burden of diabetes because everyone will make adjustments to it in some way. Because diabetes is the second most common chronic disease in children after asthma, the whole family needs to work together to make living with the disease as easy as possible.

In this chapter, you find out how to manage diabetes in your child at each stage of growth and development. You need to remember that your child is first a child and then a child with diabetes. And you also need to remember that you're not to blame for your child's diabetes. It's also important to remember that your child is not to blame either.

Caring for Your Baby or Preschooler

Your baby can't tell you what's bothering him. For this reason, as parents, you may miss the fact that he's urinating excessively in his nappy. He'll lose weight and have vomiting and diarrhoea, but this may be described as a stomach disorder rather than diabetes. When the diagnosis is finally made, your baby may be very sick and may require a stay in a paediatric intensive care unit or ward. Do not blame yourself for not realising that your baby was sick.

Once the diagnosis is made, the hard work begins. You need to learn to give insulin injections and to test the blood glucose in a child who will be reluctant to have either one done. You have to learn when and what to feed your baby, both to encourage growth and development and to prevent low blood glucose.

At this stage, you're not as worried about tight control as you will be later on. There are several reasons for this. Firstly, your baby's neurological system is still developing; frequent, severe low blood glucose will damage this development, so the glucose is permitted to be higher now than later on. Secondly, studies show that changes associated with high blood glucose leading to complications do not begin to add up until the prepubescent years, so you have a grace period during which you can exercise less tight control.

Even though you can allow blood glucose to be higher now than later on, a small baby is very fragile. There is less of everything, so small losses of water, sodium, potassium and other substances will more rapidly lead to a very sick baby. If you keep your baby's blood glucose around 5 to 12 mmol/L, you're doing very well.

For a time of variable duration, as your infant grows, your child will have seemingly regained the ability to control the blood glucose with little or no insulin, the so-called honeymoon period (see the sidebar 'The honeymoon period' later in this chapter). This period always ends.

When the honeymoon ends, you have to work with the doctor, the dietitian and the diabetes educator to find out how to control diabetes with insulin. You need to know how to do the following:

- Identify the signs and symptoms of hyperglycaemia (high blood sugar levels, hypoglycaemia and diabetic ketoacidosis. See Chapter 6)

- Administer insulin (see Chapter 10)

- Measure the blood glucose and blood or urine ketones (see Chapter 9)

✔ Treat hypoglycaemia with food or glucagon (see Chapter 6)

✔ Ensure your child with diabetes receives proper nutrition (see Chapter 11)

✔ Know what to do when your child is sick with another childhood illness (see the section 'Caring for a Sick Child' later in this chapter)

Your responsibilities as the parent of a baby with diabetes are extensive and time-consuming. Training your usual helpers to take over, even for a short time, is especially difficult. Unless you hire a professional to take over for a while, you may not get very much time away from an infant who has diabetes.

Your other children may resent the attention that you give this one child; if they start to misbehave, this resentment may be the reason. Try to work as a team and involve the whole family when making decisions. The social worker or psychologist in your diabetes care team can be of great help in this situation.

If diabetes occurs in a preschooler, the diagnosis may present similar challenges to those that arise when diabetes is diagnosed in a baby. If a honeymoon period occurs after the diagnosis, this period is usually briefer than if a diagnosis is made in a teenager.

The honeymoon period

Called the 'honeymoon period' because it represents a period of improvement in type 1 diabetes that does not last, the honeymoon period does occur in most patients.

Once the diagnosis has been made and the condition has been treated so that the blood glucose levels are close to normal, your child may require little or no insulin for a time. This is a period of remission in the disease and means some function in the beta cells of the pancreas still exists (refer to Chapter 3). Longer remissions are seen when

✔ The age at onset of diabetes is older.

✔ The initial presentation of the disease is milder.

✔ The level of islet cell antibodies is lower (refer to Chapter 3).

This remission is temporary and ends with a sudden or slowly increasing requirement for insulin. By three years after the diagnosis, complete loss of insulin production in young children is apparent. Older children may have some preservation of function.

Preschoolers are beginning the process of separating from their parents and starting to learn to control their environment (by becoming toilet-trained, for example). This separation process makes it more difficult for you, the parent, to give the injections and test the glucose. You must be firm in insisting that these things be done. You'll need to do them yourself because a small child neither knows how to do them nor understands what to do with the information generated by the glucose meter.

Because a child's eating habits may not be very regular, the use of ultra short-acting insulin or an insulin pump is especially helpful (refer to Chapter 10).

Looking After Your Primary School Child

In some ways, diabetes care gets a little easier with a primary school child, but in other ways, it gets more difficult. Your child can tell you when she has symptoms of hypoglycaemia, so this is easier to recognise and treat. However, your child is reaching the stage where control really counts, which may mean a change in or tightening of insulin therapy.

You still have a child who is growing and developing, so nutrition remains very important. Enough of the right kinds of kilojoules must be provided for this process.

As your child goes to school, she interacts with other children and wants their approval and wants to fit in. Diabetes may be considered a stigma by your child. She may be very reluctant to tell other children about it. A plan of treatment that interferes with school and friendships may be very unwelcome.

Your child is going to do more to separate from you. She may insist on giving insulin injections and doing blood tests herself. Studies again indicate that this is not a good time for you to give up these tasks, certainly not completely. Your child may not be physically capable of performing them and, in an attempt to hide the disease from peers, may not perform them at all during school hours. Diet may also suffer at school as your child tries to fit in and not stand out by eating the things that diabetes requires.

Once again the social worker or child psychologist in your diabetes care team is there to help. This person can spend time with both the child with diabetes and the family to help them develop coping strategies and provide ongoing support during difficult times.

Because you're beginning to tighten the level of control, your child has a higher risk of hypoglycaemia, especially at night. You can avoid the onset of hypoglycaemia in your child by using any or all of the following methods at this stage and from now on:

✔ Measure and treat low blood glucose before bedtime.

✔ Occasionally check the blood glucose at 3 am especially if your child has been very active that day or if her blood glucose levels were low at bedtime.

✔ Ask about symptoms of night-time low blood glucose, such as nightmares and headaches.

✔ Be sure your child does not miss meals.

✔ Have your child eat carbohydrate before exercising if the blood glucose level is less than 7 mmol/L.

✔ Reduce your child's insulin when exercising once you have spoken to your child's diabetes care team.

Some member of the family must be able to administer glucagon by injection to treat hypoglycaemia should you be unable to get the child to eat or drink. The technique for administering glucagon can be taught by your diabetes care team.

Once your child is off to school or is at day care, you need to address new problems. All staff need to know that they are caring for a child or have a student with diabetes. You need to help the staff by providing information about your child's health and needs.

The Australian Diabetes Council (in NSW), Diabetes Australia (in other states) and the Juvenile Diabetes Research Foundation Australia (JDRF) help with the needs of children and young adults with diabetes by providing information, support, counselling, advice and education for the general public to alert people to the nature of type 1 diabetes. JDRF receives little government funding and raises money particularly for research through a variety of projects. The most well known is the 'Walk for the Cure', which occurs in most capital cities every year.

Your diabetes team or the Australian Diabetes Council (in NSW) and Diabetes Australia (in other states) can arrange for an educator to visit the school and talk to teachers and other school staff members about the special requirements of children with diabetes.

Staff need to be aware of the symptoms of hypoglycaemia and how to treat it in an emergency by giving the child something sweet, such as juice (125 millilitres) or seven jellybeans, perhaps followed by a more substantial form of carbohydrate. Teachers need to be particularly watchful just before meal times or at times of increased exercise.

Often, the school will work together with the parents and their doctor to develop a management plan that must include:

- Blood glucose monitoring
- Insulin administration
- Meals and snacks
- Recognition and treatment of hypoglycaemia and hyperglycaemia

As the parent, you're responsible for providing all supplies for testing and treatment. The school has a responsibility to provide a duty of care and adequate supervision. Provision needs to be made for your child to test his blood glucose and take insulin in private. The school staff need to be able to understand and treat hypoglycaemia and understand that due to hyperglycaemia your child may need to use the toilet more frequently. Communicating well with the school is important so that school life is as uneventful as possible.

Supporting Your Adolescent

Your adolescent or teenager with diabetes will provide some of your biggest challenges. This is the time that most childhood diabetes begins. The Diabetes Control and Complications Trial showed that tight control can be accomplished beginning at age 13, and that this control can prevent complications. The higher frequency of severe hypoglycaemia that accompanies tighter control was not found to be damaging to the brain of a child at this age. However, children at this age don't think in terms of long-term blood glucose control and prevention of complications, so many are not willing to do many of the tasks required to control their diabetes on a regular basis.

The age group of your child is likely to have a significant impact on the target glycosylated HbA1c levels. Most guidelines suggest a target HbA1c of between 6.5 and 7 per cent, as long as this can be achieved without too many hypoglycaemic episodes. The International Society for Pediatric and Adolescent Diabetes (ISPAD) guidelines suggest 7.5 per cent for all age groups. Because all children are individuals, discuss and agree upon your child's target levels with your diabetes care team.

This stage is when your child will be most eager to become independent. You don't want to give up all control at this time for several reasons:

✔ Your child actually does better if he has limits that are clearly stated and enforced.

✔ Young people may find it difficult to tell their peers they have diabetes, and this may cause them to miss injections and food, especially when they are with friends.

✔ The problem of eating disorders (refer to Chapter 11) may arise at this time, especially among girls trying to maintain a slim body image. Like all people with type 1 diabetes, these girls with diabetes know that if they miss their injections, they will lose weight, and they ignore the high blood glucose that results.

✔ Teenagers with diabetes may still be unable to translate levels of blood glucose into appropriate action.

The hormonal changes that occur in puberty are often associated with insulin resistance. This is the most likely cause of loss of control rather than any failure of your child to follow the diabetes treatment plan. Upward adjustment of the insulin is usually required at this time. The young adolescent shouldn't be 'blamed' for this — it's part of growing up. The level of the blood glucose is what's important, not the amount of insulin taken.

Handing Over Control to the Young Adult

Health care needs of young adults are different to those of children and adults. As your child with diabetes becomes an older teenager, this imposes unique challenges on your child, you and your family and your diabetes team. When you hand over control and give your child more independence will vary depending on her maturity.

One sign that your child is ready to be cared for in the health system as an adult is if she is independent with all the tasks involved in diabetes care. Your diabetes care team can offer more guidance to help you work out if the time is right to move from paediatric care to an adult endocrinologist and diabetes team. This process is known as *transition* and many paediatric diabetes teams have specific transition services to facilitate a smooth move from the paediatric world to adult diabetes services.

Your child now has new challenges, including finding work, going to university, making new friends and finding a place to live independently. She should have intensive diabetes care and management at this point, which may include multiple injections or an insulin pump (refer to Chapter 10). Check out Chapter 11 for more on a suitable dietary approach when on multiple injections or a pump. Advice about exercise can be found in Chapter 12.

Helping the Obese Child with Type 2 Diabetes

The epidemic of obesity, which has spread to children in Australia in the past few decades, has led to a much higher prevalence of type 2 diabetes in children than was ever seen before. Even without diabetes, obesity is a burden for children. The obese child can have severe psychological and social problems:

- Less comfortable family interactions
- Less respect from peers than other children with disabilities receive
- Low self-esteem
- Poor body image

Adding type 2 diabetes into this mix can be devastating. The consequences of the preceding problems may lead to failure to manage the diabetes because the child wants to avoid any activity that will make him even more different from peers.

Only a fraction of overweight or obese children go on to develop diabetes, but it is important to separate type 1 diabetes from type 2 because the treatment may be quite different in type 2. The key differences that suggest a diagnosis of type 2 in children rather than type 1 are:

- A family history of type 2 diabetes
- A reserve of insulin in the body, as shown by a C-peptide level in the blood that is normal or elevated (C-peptide is made every time insulin is produced, so its presence indicates that the body is making insulin)
- A velvety darkening of the skin, especially under the arms, called *acanthosis nigricans*

✔ Belonging to certain ethnic groups such as Aboriginal Australians or Torres Strait and Pacific Islanders

✔ Extremely rare ketoacidosis (refer to Chapter 6)

✔ No evidence of autoimmunity (refer to Chapter 3)

✔ Obesity

The child with type 2 diabetes has a different type of diabetes and can be treated with tablets or diet and exercise alone. However, because children often don't appreciate long-term consequences of their actions, you often have the problem of compliance.

You must help your obese child to lose weight because many obese children will become obese adults. With the assistance of a dietitian, you can work out the food that your child can eat to maintain growth and development without further weight gain. If your child is old enough, one of the most helpful techniques is to take the child into the supermarket and point out healthy food choices. It may also be helpful to keep problem foods out of the house, so there is much less likelihood that your child will eat them. Regular physical activity — be it joining a sporting team, dancing, swimming or playing in the park — will be of great help to the child with type 2 diabetes.

As parents, you should try to offer good role models to your children when it comes to lifestyle changes. Kids love to mirror adult behaviour, so if they see you eating healthily and exercising regularly, this will help them to appreciate the value of these activities.

Caring for a Sick Child

Your child is susceptible to all the usual childhood illnesses, but diabetes can complicate your management. An illness can affect diabetes in varied ways. An infection may increase the level of insulin resistance so that the usual dose of insulin is not adequate. Or it may cause nausea and vomiting so that no food or drink can stay down, and the insulin may cause hypoglycaemia. For this reason, you need to measure the blood glucose in your sick child every two hours and call a diabetes educator or doctor if you observe an increase in levels over time. If the glucose is over 15 mmol/L, you need to give extra rapid-acting insulin. The dose required is usually about 10 to 20 per cent of the total daily insulin dose.

If the blood glucose levels are over 15 mmol/L, ketones should be tested in the urine or blood (refer to Chapter 9). If these levels become elevated, you need to discuss the situation with your diabetes care team or implement the sick day plan you have developed with the team.

For a more detailed discussion of creating a plan for sick days, refer to Chapter 6.

You should probably feed your child with clear liquids like diet cordial and diet lemonade during the sick days if blood sugar levels are high. If your child has a stomach upset, milk may be excluded because it may make things worse. As long as your child can hold down clear liquids, you can continue to take care of her. If clear liquids cannot be held down, you must contact your GP or diabetes care team and take your child to the hospital.

While the blood glucose remains over 12 mmol/L, use water and diet soft drinks so as not to add carbohydrates. When the blood glucose is less than 12 mmol/L, you can use regular soft drinks or glucose drinks. But remember — please call your doctor or diabetes educator for help.

Liaising with Your Diabetes Care Team

Especially when your child is first diagnosed with diabetes, the stress can be overwhelming. The guilt that comes with this diagnosis may leave you unable to help your child much at first and certainly unable to learn all that you need to know to master all of the areas of importance to the health of your child. This is when you must depend upon the help of the diabetes care team, more at the beginning, but throughout the duration of his childhood.

The diabetes educator will show you how to administer insulin and test the blood glucose. The educator will also explain how to use the information to determine an insulin dose. The dietitian can explain about carbohydrate exchanges and healthy food choices for growth and development (refer to Chapter 11). The diabetes educator can explain the short- and long-term complications of diabetes and how your child can avoid them. The social worker or psychologist can help you deal with the psychological issues at each stage of your child's development. One of these people can also help you with an exercise program for your child.

One resource that can be tremendously valuable for you and your child is the diabetes camps run by organisations affiliated with the Australian Diabetes Council (in NSW), Diabetes Australia (in other states or territories) or the Juvenile Diabetes Research Foundation Australia (JDFR). These camps are located all over the country and provide a safe, well-managed place where your child can go and be in the majority. Children can learn a great deal about diabetes while enjoying all the pleasures of a camp environment. (Certainly not a minor benefit is the opportunity for you to have time off for perhaps the first time in years.)

You can find out more about camps for children with diabetes throughout Australia by contacting the Australian Diabetes Council (in NSW), Diabetes Australia (in other states or territories) or JDRF and they will put you in touch with camping organisations in your state or territory. See Chapter 24 for website details for these organisations.

In Chapter 14, we compare diabetes to a stage play. There, the person with diabetes is the author, the producer, the director and the star. When you have a child with diabetes, your child is the star, but you take on the roles of author, producer and director. You obviously have a great responsibility but one that we feel certain you can handle. You don't need to do it alone. Use your medical experts as well as your family and friends to make it manageable.

Chapter 17

Diabetes and the Older Person

· ·

In This Chapter

▶ Detecting diabetes in older people

▶ Considering intellectual functioning

▶ Dealing with dietary considerations

▶ Focusing on the unique eye problems of the older person

▶ Solving urinary and sexual problems

▶ Considering the best treatment option for the individual

· ·

*E*veryone wants to live a long time, but no-one wants to get old. Nevertheless, getting old is better than the alternative. Woody Allen says the one advantage of dying is that you don't have to do jury duty. We'd rather do jury duty.

Defining 'the older person' is the first problem. Every year the definition seems to change, but we think it's fair to talk about the age of 65 as the beginning of 'older'. By that definition, by the year 2020, the number of older people in Australia is predicted to increase by approximately 50 per cent on current numbers. It is also predicted that by 2020 the number of older people will outnumber those under the age of 25. A recent study showed that about 18 per cent of the older population have diabetes and a further 11 per cent have impaired glucose tolerance. Between 1995 and 2004, the overall prevalence of diabetes in the older person increased by 7 per cent.

Older people with diabetes have special problems. They're hospitalised at a much higher rate than the general population of older people. Even without hospitalisation, older people with diabetes have special problems. In this chapter, you find out about those problems and the way to handle them.

Diagnosing Diabetes in the Older Person

The incidence of diabetes in the older person is higher for many reasons, but the main culprit seems to be increasing insulin resistance with ageing, even if the older person with diabetes is not particularly obese or sedentary. Doctors don't yet understand why insulin resistance increases. When they look at the pancreas, it seems to be able to make insulin at the usual rate. The fasting blood glucose actually rises very slowly as you get older. It's the glucose after meals that rises much quicker and leads to the diagnosis. Between normal and the value that indicates diabetes is a grey zone that is probably impaired glucose tolerance (refer to Chapter 5).

What seems to happen with increasing age is that the pancreas 'tires out' and produces less insulin. Older individuals sometimes have the combined problem of *insulin resistance* (insulin not working) and *insulin deficiency* (not enough insulin). That leads to the need of insulin therapy in some older people.

Older people with diabetes often don't complain of any symptoms. When they do, the symptoms may not be the ones usually associated with type 2 diabetes or they may be confusing. Older people with diabetes may complain of loss of appetite or weakness, and they may have lost weight rather than become obese. They may have incontinence of urine, which is usually thought of as a prostate problem in men or a urinary tract infection in women. Older people with diabetes may not complain of thirst because their ability to feel thirst is altered.

Evaluating Intellectual Functioning

Evaluating the intellectual function of an older person with diabetes is good to do from time to time because management of the disease requires a fairly high level of mental functioning. The patient has to follow a healthy diet, administer medications properly and test the blood glucose on a regular basis. Studies have shown that older people with diabetes have a higher incidence of *dementia* (loss of mental functioning) and Alzheimer's disease than older people without diabetes, making it much harder for them to perform these self-care activities. However, by detecting a problem early, strategies can be put in place to assist older people in continuing to care for themselves.

The doctor can administer *cognitive screening tests* to determine the level of function. Testing makes it easier to tell whether the patient can be self-sufficient or will need help. Many older people with diabetes living alone with no assistance may require an assisted-living situation or even an aged care facility.

In Australia, you can ask your local Aged Care Assessment Team (ACAT) to provide a full assessment of an older person. If help is required to keep someone at home or if the person requires transfer to an aged care facility, the ACAT team can assist in organising both options. Government subsidies for home care services are available to help older people stay in their own homes as long as possible.

Reconsidering Dietary Restrictions

In addition to the intellectual function required to understand and prepare a healthy diet (see the preceding section), as people age they may have other problems when it comes to proper nutrition:

- ✔ They may have poor vision and be unable to see to read or cook.
- ✔ They may be on a low income and be unable to purchase the foods that they require.
- ✔ Their senses of taste and smell may be decreased, so they lose interest in food.
- ✔ They often have a loss of appetite.
- ✔ They may have arthritis or a tremor that prevents them preparing and cooking food.
- ✔ They may have poor teeth or a dry mouth.

Any one of these problems may be enough to prevent proper eating by the older person with the result that the diabetes is poorly controlled. They may also be malnourished, even if their weight appears normal or even if they are overweight, as the quality of the diet is so poor.

It's hard to imagine, but the older person still needs a diet rich in nutrients not unlike a teenager, even if the required kilojoule intake is less. However, the challenge is trying to achieve these requirements when appetite may have diminished or functional ability declines.

Your specialist diabetes dietitian can help you address the dietary challenges faced by an older person with diabetes, and develop strategies with you to improve day-to-day life. For example, your dietitan can help you set up Meals on Wheels visits, or provide advice about meals that are nutritious but easy to prepare.

Dealing with Eye Problems

Older people with diabetes have the eye problems that are brought on by diabetes earlier, and they can affect all aspects of proper diabetes care. They may develop cataracts, macular degeneration and open angle glaucoma in addition to diabetic retinopathy. (Refer to Chapter 7 for more information on these eye problems.)

One of the biggest failures in diabetes care is that as many as one-third of older people never have an eye examination at all. How can disease be found when it's early enough to treat if no examination is done?

Once these problems are detected, they can be treated and vision saved.

Make sure you have a proper eye examination every year! In Australia, many optometrists can now screen for diabetic eye disease and seeing an optometrist is Medicare-funded. (Refer to Chapter 14 for more on eye testing.)

Coping with Urinary and Sexual Problems

Urinary and sexual problems are very common in older people with diabetes and can greatly affect quality of life. It's not uncommon for an older person with diabetes to have paralysis of the bladder muscle with retention of urine followed by overflow incontinence when the bladder fills up. An older person may be unable to get to the toilet fast enough. Sometimes spasms in the bladder muscle lead to incontinence. The result may be frequent urinary tract infections.

Almost 60 per cent of men over the age of 70 are impotent, and 50 per cent have no *libido*, a desire to have sex. These problems can have many causes (refer to Chapter 7), but older men are especially likely to have blockage of blood vessels with poor flow into the penis. Older Australians take an average of seven medications daily, many of which can also affect sexual function.

To have sex at any age, you need sexual desire and the physical ability to perform, you need a willing partner, and you need a safe, private place. Any or all of these may be missing for the older person.

It's not always necessary to treat sexual dysfunction if the person with diabetes and that person's partner are okay with the situation as it is. If not, Chapter 7 points out a number of treatments for sexual problems.

Designing an Appropriate Treatment Program

When deciding upon treatment, you first have to consider your goals. Do you have a very elderly person with diabetes with a low life expectancy, or do you have a person with diabetes who is older but physiologically young and could live for 15 or 20 more years? A person who has lived to age 65 has a life expectancy of at least 18 more years, plenty of time to develop complications of diabetes, especially macrovascular disease, eye disease, kidney disease and nervous system disease (refer to Chapter 7).

Choosing the best blood glucose target

In the past, most doctors believed that the more they could keep a patient's blood glucose within the normal range, the better as it would prevent long-term complications of diabetes. While this is true for some complications (especially eye disease and kidney disease), no strong evidence exists that the intensive-care approach prevents complications such as heart attacks and stroke.

The benefit of the intensive approach must be balanced against the risk of hypoglycaemia. This is especially important in older people, where very low glucose levels, which can lead to falls and fainting, can be dangerous.

In the older person, it's important to strike a balance. Blood glucose levels should be controlled but not at the expense of frequent hypoglycaemia. Older people should have regular meals and be familiar with the symptoms and treatment of hypoglycaemia (refer to Chapter 6).

Looking at diet, exercise and medication

Treatment of diabetes always starts with diet and exercise, but exercise may be limited in the older person with diabetes. Of course, exercise is helpful, even in the very old, as recent studies have shown. Exercise reduces the blood glucose and the glycosylated HbA1c. However, because older people may have more coronary artery disease, arthritis, eye disease, neuropathy and peripheral vascular disease, exercise just may not be possible. (Refer to Chapter 12 for more on exercise.)

The diet for the older person with diabetes is basically the same as that for the younger person with diabetes. However, when you're older you can be as much at risk for malnutrition as for obesity, and a very strict, low-fat diet may no longer be required. A balanced approach is usually the best option — your specialist diabetes dietitian can help with a diet reassessment and with healthy eating tips for the older person. (Refer to the section 'Reconsidering Dietary Restrictions', earlier in this chapter, and Chapter 11.)

Education for the patient who can benefit can be of great value, especially if the partner is also involved.

If medications must be added, this can be complicated by a number of considerations particular to the older person:

- The person may not be able to see the correct dosage.
- The person may be mentally unable to take the medicine properly.
- Physical limitations may prevent medication taking, especially insulin.
- Multiple other drugs may interact with the diabetes medicine.
- Older people have decreased kidney and liver function, making some drugs for diabetes last longer.
- Poor nutrition may make them more prone to hypoglycaemia.

We explain medication usage in Chapter 10, but, again, drugs in the older person must be handled more carefully. Of the sulphonylurea drugs, chlorpropamide is the longest acting and can cause very prolonged hypoglycaemia, so it's not used often after the age of 65. Most doctors use the newer sulphonylureas like glipizide and gliclazide.

Metformin can lower the blood glucose without the fear of hypoglycaemia and can be very useful in the older population for this reason. It often causes weight loss, which may be helpful for many patients, but we have seen it cause very excessive weight loss in certain more elderly people. Because older people have diminished kidney function, metformin must be used with care and not used at all when alcoholism, liver disease or acute infection exists.

Pioglitazone belongs to a group of drugs that may reverse the process — insulin resistance — that makes diabetes so prevalent in older people. While rosiglitazone, a related drug, is much less used nowadays, due to its potential effects on the heart, pioglitazone continues to be a medication option for the older person. Another advantage of pioglitazone is that it doesn't cause hypoglycaemia.

Pioglitazone must be used cautiously in an older person with heart problems, as the medication can make symptoms of some heart conditions (such as heart failure) worse.

New therapies such as exenatide (Byetta) and sitagliptin (Januvia) (discussed in Chapter 10) may have an increasing role in the older person. These medications don't cause hypoglycaemia and may lead to weight loss. Similar to metformin, they should be used with care in an older person with kidney disease.

Insulin is added when the oral drugs have failed. For basic treatment, a night-time injection of long-acting insulin like glargine (Lantus), along with daytime tablets, may be all that is needed. For intensive treatment, two daily injections of a premixed insulin or multiple injections of intermediate and rapid-acting insulin will be needed, along with frequent monitoring of the blood glucose. (Refer to Chapter 10 for more information on insulin.) This level of treatment may be hard to accomplish with a very elderly patient who is not in an aged care facility.

The ability of the person to cope with the different strategies required should be taken into consideration when an insulin regime is prescribed by a diabetes care team. Diabetes educators and doctors work together closely to ensure the right regimen is suggested.

A patient who is transferred from self-care to institutional care may require a change in medication because he may not have been taking the medication properly at home or may now be eating differently. The diabetes care team should be involved during these times of change to assist the person with diabetes to achieve the health care targets required.

Chapter 18

Diabetes and Pregnancy

· ·

In This Chapter

▶ Avoiding pregnancy problems when you have diabetes prior to pregnancy

▶ Ensuring mother and baby stay well through a diabetic pregnancy

▶ Keeping an eye on baby after birth and starting breastfeeding

▶ Monitoring blood glucose after pregnancy

· ·

*P*regnancy in a mother with diabetes is definitely more complicated than in a mother without diabetes. For this reason, clinics around the country employ the latest techniques and equipment, and knowledgeable health care workers are available for consultation.

If you have diabetes and want to become pregnant, you need to be reviewed by your diabetes specialist before you conceive.

About 0.4 per cent of pregnancies occur in women with pre-existing diabetes, called *pregestational diabetes,* and an additional 3 to 7 per cent occur in women who develop diabetes some time in the second half of the pregnancy, called *gestational diabetes.*

With the proper precautions, the diabetic pregnancy can proceed like a pregnancy without diabetes. This chapter describes everything you need to know to enjoy a healthy pregnancy and deliver a healthy baby.

Pregnancy and Pregestational Diabetes

In a non-diabetic pregnancy, the body makes enough insulin to overcome the effect of pregnancy hormones (which block insulin action) and the blood glucose stays normal. A woman with type 1 diabetes can't make more insulin and needs two or three times the usual dose. The increasing need for insulin usually stabilises in the last several weeks of the pregnancy and by the last one or two weeks, you may begin to have hypoglycaemia. Once the baby and placenta are delivered, your insulin needs are reduced immediately.

A woman with type 1 diabetes may have some retinopathy (damage to the back of the eye — refer to Chapter 7). If this is present, it needs to be treated and stabilised before conception as it may deteriorate during pregnancy. This deterioration is probably the result of rapid improvement of the blood glucose in a woman who has been poorly controlled previously. Once the pregnancy is completed, the eyes will return to their previous state.

Kidney disease (refer to Chapter 7) increases the risk of pre-eclampsia (elevated blood pressure, fluid retention and protein in the urine). Severe, permanent worsening of the kidney disease is unusual, but a temporary decline in kidney function may occur.

If you have type 1 diabetes, you must take action in advance to avoid the problems of pregnancy by controlling your glucose before conception. (See Part III for information on how to manage your diabetes.) Tighter blood glucose control may be achieved by using an insulin pump, which has been proved to be safe to continue using during pregnancy. Speak with your diabetes care team if you wish to consider pump use prior to conception.

Like all pregnant women, those with diabetes need to ensure that their dietary intakes are adequate for pregnancy, especially in the last trimester (or final three months). This is in addition to the dietary care they may be taking to manage their blood glucose levels. (See the section 'Treating diabetes in pregnancy' later in this chapter for more information.)

Like those with pre-existing type 1 diabetes, a woman with type 2 diabetes can certainly become pregnant; however, she must discuss her pregnancy plans with her GP or diabetes care team, as good control is important at conception. Waiting until after conception to improve diabetes control is too late as damage may have already been done to the tiny foetus.

If you are on oral agents to lower glucose, you may need to stop them and use insulin to control the glucose. In addition, obesity, a frequent finding in type 2 diabetes, puts the person at greater risk of hypertension during the pregnancy. Evaluation of the type 2 patient is similar to that of the type 1 patient. Most of these pregnancies can be allowed to go to term, but if the woman is suffering from hypertension or has had a previous complicated delivery, then earlier delivery needs to be considered.

Managing a Diabetic Pregnancy

In Australia, all pregnant women are screened for gestational diabetes, meaning all women who developed diabetes through the course of their pregnancy will be identified. As well as all the other factors that need to be kept in mind when a woman is pregnant, women with gestational or pregestational diabetes are presented with a whole new set of considerations when it comes to caring for themselves and their babies. This section covers all these considerations, from diagnosis to delivery.

Diagnosing diabetes in pregnant women

Experts disagree as to whether all pregnant women who don't already have diabetes need to be checked for it. Some advocate selective screening, suggesting that a thin pregnant woman with no family history of diabetes who is physically active is an unlikely candidate for diabetes. However, the current consensus is to screen all women because a small but significant number of patients with gestational diabetes will be missed if all women are not screened. Everyone agrees that if the glucose tolerance is normal in weeks 27 to 31 of the pregnancy, you don't need to do more screening. If gestational diabetes was present in a previous pregnancy or the women are in another high-risk group (such as Aboriginal Australians, certain ethnic groups, women who have previously given birth to a baby over 4.5 kilograms or women who are hypertensive), the screening test is done as early as the 13th week.

The screening test (non-fasting modified glucose tolerance test) is done between weeks 26 and 28 of the pregnancy. No preparation is necessary. You consume a drink containing 50 grams of glucose, and a blood glucose level is obtained from a vein before the drink and again at one hour after consumption. If the glucose level one hour after the drink is less than 7.8 mmol/L, it's considered normal. If it's greater than 7.8 mmol/L, a further test is done to make a diagnosis of gestational diabetes, because many women who have a value greater than 7.8 mmol/L will not necessarily have diabetes.

The definitive test (fasting oral glucose tolerance test) is done as follows:

 ✓ The woman prepares by eating at least 200 grams of carbohydrate daily for three days and fasting for at least eight hours before the test.

 ✓ The woman consumes a drink containing 75 grams of glucose.

✔ Blood glucose is measured before the glucose drink, at one and again at two hours after ingestion of the glucose.

✔ A diagnosis of gestational diabetes is made if the initial blood glucose level (fasting) is greater than 5.5 mmol/L and the two-hour blood glucose level is greater than 8 mmol/L.

The preceding list shows the current criteria for making the diagnosis of gestational diabetes from the Australian Diabetes in Pregnancy Society (ADIPS). However, these criteria may change if new International Association of the Diabetes and Pregnancy Study Groups (IADPSG) criteria are adopted. You can find further information on these criteria on the ADIPS website (www.adips.org) or from your endocrinologist.

Coping with diabetes and pregnancy

If a woman is found to have gestational diabetes or already has pregestational diabetes, a whole new group of considerations arise in order to deliver a healthy baby while maintaining the health of the mother. Blood glucose levels, blood pressure and weight gain need to be carefully monitored throughout the pregnancy to ensure target levels are being met and maintained.

A high blood glucose left untreated has major consequences for mother and foetus. If present early in the pregnancy, the result may be *congenital malformations* (physical abnormalities that may be life threatening) in the foetus. In the third trimester, the growing foetus may exhibit *macrosomia* (abnormal largeness) that can lead to a too-early delivery, or damage to the baby or mother during delivery of the very large baby.

Measuring the risks

The HbA1c is an excellent measurement of overall glucose control and provides a good indicator for the risk of miscarriage or risk of foetal abnormalities.

If it is high, it indicates that the woman with diabetes was in poor control at conception, and the likelihood of a miscarriage and/or congenital problems is greater. If overall glucose control is normal the risk of miscarriage is no more likely than that in a woman without diabetes.

The situation for congenital malformations is a little more complicated. Such malformations increase with increasing glucose as well, but also with the level of *ketones,* the breakdown product of fats. However, measuring the ketones will not tell you if malformations will definitely occur. (Refer to Chapter 9 for more on measuring ketones.)

Babies where only the father has diabetes develop normally. The environment in which the foetus is developing, not the genetic material provided by the father, is responsible for the potential abnormalities in a pregnancy complicated by diabetes. Elevated blood glucose, any abnormalities of proteins and fats that result from the elevated glucose, and the loss of sensitivity to insulin explain the problems which may occur in pregnancies where diabetes is diagnosed in the mother.

Early pregnancy problems

The major concern of the woman with pregestational diabetes is to have good blood glucose control at the time of conception.

Both miscarriages and congenital malformations can be a result of poor glucose control at conception and/or shortly thereafter. The woman with diabetes who wants to become pregnant must be in good control before she attempts to become pregnant to prevent these problems from occurring. High blood glucose levels can induce foetal malformations. (For more on managing diabetes, see Part III.)

However, a woman in poor control of her diabetes has more trouble conceiving a baby than a woman who is in good control, which may be the major reason that more babies aren't born with congenital malformations. If you're concerned about your level of control prior to becoming pregnant, see your diabetes care team for help and advice to get yourself back on track.

A woman who has gestational diabetes doesn't have to worry that her baby is more likely to have congenital malformations than babies whose mothers don't have diabetes. This is because her blood glucose didn't start to rise until halfway through the pregnancy, long after the baby's important body structures were formed.

Late pregnancy problems

Women with both pregestational and gestational diabetes need to be concerned about delivering a large baby. This largeness is not proportional — this is, the areas that are most responsive to insulin, where fat is stored in the baby, are the ones that enlarge the most.

A baby is considered large if it weighs more than 4.5 kilograms at birth. Most large babies are the offspring of mothers without diabetes. Their growth is proportional throughout the pregnancy so that their shoulders are not out of proportion to their heads, and delivery is not as complicated.

Why macrosomia occurs

Macrosomia, or a large baby, that can occur with pregestational or gestational diabetes has to do with the elevated glucose, fat and amino acid levels in the mother in the second half of pregnancy. If these levels aren't lowered, the foetus is exposed to high levels of these nutrients. This stimulates the foetal pancreas to begin to make insulin earlier and to store these extra nutrients as body fat.

The foetus becomes large wherever fat is stored, such as the shoulders, chest, abdomen, arms and legs. Because they are large, these macrosomic babies are delivered early in order to make the delivery easier and avoid birth trauma. However, though they are large, they may not be fully mature. This predisposes these babies to the risk of respiratory distress.

Treating diabetes in pregnancy

This section covers all aspects of a diabetic pregnancy, for women with either pregestational or gestational diabetes.

Pregnancy and type 1 diabetes

In addition to controlling your glucose levels before conceiving, the pregestational woman with diabetes needs to do the following:

- ✔ Use contraception to plan the timing of conception to ensure your blood glucose levels are optimal at and after conception
- ✔ Check immunity for rubella and chickenpox
- ✔ Discontinue prescription drugs that harm a foetus (check with your GP for details)
- ✔ Have your eyes and kidneys checked to establish a baseline for future damage control
- ✔ Stop tobacco and alcohol use
- ✔ Take a 5 milligram folate supplement each day
- ✔ Meet with your diabetes care team to plan care

If you're a pregestational woman with diabetes, you need to achieve a stricter level of control during pregnancy than when you aren't pregnant. Your foetus is removing glucose from you at a rapid rate, so your blood glucose level is lower than usual. In addition, your body turns to fat for fuel much sooner, so you produce ketones earlier. Too many ketones can damage the foetus as well. The fact that you break down fat so early is termed *accelerated starvation*.

In order to maintain your blood glucose at the proper level, you must measure it more frequently. You should measure it before meals, at bedtime and one hour after eating. Your goal is to achieve the levels of blood glucose listed in Table 18-1.

Table 18-1	Optimum Levels of Blood Glucose	
Fasting and Pre-meal	*1 Hour After*	*2 Hours After*
Less than 5 mmol/L	Less than 8 mmol/L	Less than 7 mmol/L

Studies have shown that the one-hour-after-meal glucose may be the most important for the pregnant woman with diabetes to keep under control. Some women may prefer to use an insulin pump (see Appendix A) to achieve the very tight control required for pregnancy. Consult with your diabetes care team if considering insulin pump therapy.

You also need to measure the level of ketones, particularly if you are unwell. Ketones can be checked by blood or urine. (Refer to Chapter 9 for more on ketone testing.) If the test is positive, it means that you're not eating enough carbohydrates, and your body is going into accelerated starvation. Too much of this condition is not good for the growing foetus.

Diet and diabetes while pregnant

The appropriate amount of weight gain during pregnancy depends upon your weight at the time you become pregnant. If your body mass index (BMI) is normal (refer to Chapter 11), you should gain 11 to 16 kilograms during the pregnancy. However, if you are overweight, then you need to gain less weight during pregnancy — that is, between 7 and 11 kilograms. If you're obese, you should gain no more than 9 kilograms. Regular visits to the dietitan during the pregnancy can help you keep your weight gain under control.

Chapter 11 tells you what you need to know about diet and diabetes. As a pregnant woman with diabetes, you have some special requirements:

 ✔ **Take an adequate intake of calcium.** This is most important in the final three months of the pregnancy, when the baby's bones are becoming stronger. You need 1,000 milligrams of calcium per day, or four serves of calcium-rich foods, during this trimester. One serve of calcium-rich food equals 300 millilitres of milk, a 200-gram tub of yoghurt or 40 grams of cheese.

✔ **Take an adequate intake of iron.** Many women require an iron supplement during pregnancy. Discuss getting your iron levels tested and whether you might need an iron supplement with your doctor or midwife.

✔ **Eat three meals a day plus a bedtime snack.** This helps prevent the accelerated starvation that results from the prolonged fast between dinner and breakfast. Many pregnant women also require mid-morning and/or mid-afternoon snacks, especially as the pregnancy progresses. If unsure, discuss this with your doctor or dietitian.

✔ **Maintain the fasting and pre-meal glucose at less than 5 mmol/L.** Your glucose should be less than 8 mmol/L one hour after meals.

✔ **If you have pregestational diabetes, you should see a dietitian prior to pregnancy and at least once during each trimester of your pregnancy.**

✔ **If you develop gestational diabetes, you should see a dietitian within one week of diagnosis and at least three times during the remainder of the pregnancy.**

✔ **Check your iodine intake.** A recent focus has been on ensuring pregnant women have an adequate intake of iodine during their pregnancy. The best sources of iodine are seafood and iodised salt. If your intake of these foods is at all irregular, you should discuss this with your doctor or midwife, because you may need to take a supplement.

In addition, you require a daily 5 milligram folate supplement three months prior to conception; this should be continued during the first four months of your pregnancy. This supplement has been shown to reduce the risks of having a baby with a neural tube defect (spina bifida). A moderate amount of exercise is also very helpful in controlling the blood glucose and keeping the mother in top shape during the pregnancy.

In general, most women don't need to take a multivitamin and mineral supplement before or during pregnancy. However, specific supplementation of key nutrients may be required. If in doubt, discuss with your doctor or dietitian.

If you are planning a baby after having gestational diabetes during a previous pregnancy, see a dietitian before conception, while still in the planning stages.

Avoiding harmful bacteria while pregnant

An important nutritional aspect all women should be aware of in pregnancy is the need to avoid food-borne bacteria such as listeria. This type of bacteria can cause food poisoning that may be particularly harmful to unborn babies. To reduce your risk of developing *listeriosis* (the disease caused by exposure to listeria bacteria) you should avoid the following:

- Pate
- Pre-prepared salads, such as those from salad bars and supermarkets
- Raw or smoked seafood, such as the seafood in some sushi or smoked salmon
- Ready-cooked chicken (whole or sliced) or cold meat, such as those from super-markets and sandwich bars
- Soft or unpasteurised cheeses, such as brie, camembert and ricotta

General food hygiene principles should also be followed — and should be continued once the new baby comes along. Get into practice now!

You should always:

- Cook all meat and other raw food of animal origin thoroughly
- Keep hot foods hot and cold foods cold — never lukewarm
- Keep raw foods covered and separated in your fridge
- Refrigerate food immediately after cooking and use or discard within 24 hours
- Reheat leftovers until steaming hot
- Thaw frozen food in the fridge
- Wash fruit and vegetables before consumption
- Wash hands, knives and chopping boards before preparing or cooking food

Remember: If in doubt, chuck it out!

Testing for abnormalities and getting ready for labour

A blood test called a serum alpha-fetoprotein can be done at 15 weeks of the pregnancy to determine whether neural tube defects exist in the foetus. At 18 weeks, an ultrasound can show any malformations of the growing foetus. An ultrasound, conducted by directing a sound at the foetus and catching it as it bounces back to the machine, produces a picture of the foetus that shows the presence of any abnormalities. This harmless test is not painful for the mother or the foetus.

If you have gestational diabetes, you need not worry about congenital malformations in your baby but need to avoid macrosomia (described in 'Coping with diabetes and pregnancy' earlier in this chapter). You need to follow the same dietary prescription as a pregestational woman with diabetes, and you may need to inject insulin if your fasting blood glucose is greater than 5.0 mmol/L. Oral antidiabetes agents (refer to Chapter 10) may be used at the discretion of your doctor. If you're taking insulin, you will stop it at the time of delivery because blood glucose levels will return to normal.

Early ultrasound is not necessary for a woman with gestational diabetes unless her doctor suspects that the diabetes was actually there much earlier. An ultrasound between weeks 32 and 34 can show whether foetal macrosomia exists. If macrosomia is present, then the doctor will probably perform a caesarean section, where the baby is removed through an incision made in the abdominal wall and the uterus.

It is best to deliver the baby at the end of 39 weeks when it has had a chance to mature completely. If the mother does not go into labour spontaneously, the obstetrician usually induces labour.

If you have gestational diabetes and have been taking insulin, blood glucose monitoring needs to continue after delivery. Your blood glucose is maintained after birth at 3.8 to 7.8 mmol/L with insulin, if necessary. If blood glucose levels don't return to normal levels, insulin may need to be continued.

For women with type 1 diabetes, insulin requirements are usually decreased soon after the birth.

Getting to the birthing suite

Most women with diabetes go into labour spontaneously and are able to have a vaginal birth. If you don't go into spontaneous labour, an induction of labour may occur. This can be performed in several ways:

- ✔ Balloon
- ✔ Breaking of the waters
- ✔ Gel induction
- ✔ Oxytocin

However, some women require a *lower segment caesarean section* (C-section), particularly if the baby is large or in distress. Discuss the possibility of a C-section or labour being induced with your diabetes team and obstetrician, because this will need to be planned for towards the end of your pregnancy.

For further information on what to expect during delivery, as well as tips for before and after birth, see www.diabetesvic.org.au/living-with-diabetes/pregnancy. For general information about pregnancy, labour and caring for your baby after birth, see *Pregnancy For Dummies*, 2nd Australian Edition, by Jane Palmer, Joanne Stone, Keith Eddleman and Mary Duenwald (Wiley Publishing Australia Pty Ltd).

Managing blood glucose during labour

Because your blood system is directly connected to that of your baby, it is important to control your blood glucose levels during labour to provide your baby with the best blood glucose levels at birth.

Women with type 1 diabetes and those on high doses of insulin for gestational diabetes will require an intravenous insulin infusion throughout labour to help regulate blood glucose levels.

Other observations such as blood pressure and baby's heart rate will be monitored. Progress of labour is observed by abdominal palpation and vaginal examination.

Caring for the Baby After Birth

The understanding of diabetes and pregnancy has resulted in a great reduction in malformations in these babies as well as the macrosomia that leads to complications at delivery. Unfortunately, many women with diabetes don't have tight control at conception, so an incidence of malformations still occurs. If an obvious malformation is present at birth, it's important to search for other malformations.

Other problems can occur because the foetus was producing a lot of insulin to handle all the maternal glucose entering through the placenta. Suddenly, maternal glucose is cut off at delivery, but the high levels of foetal insulin continue for a while, which can cause hypoglycaemia.

One way to reduce the risk of your baby developing hypoglycaemia is to breastfeed, which also provides other important nutrients and helps your baby build his or her immunity.

Checking for hypoglycaemia and other problems after birth

The danger of hypoglycaemia exists in the first four to six hours after delivery. The baby may be sweaty and appear nervous or even have a seizure. Frequent testing of the baby's blood glucose levels is required until he or she is stable, and then at intervals for the first 24 hours.

Besides hypoglycaemia, the baby may have several other complications right after birth:

- **Hyperbilirubinaemia (typically seen as jaundice):** This condition is the product of too much breakdown of red blood cells. It is treated with light.

- **Lazy left colon:** Occurring for unknown reasons, this condition presents itself like an obstruction of the bowel but clears up on its own.

- **Low calcium with jitteriness and possibly seizures:** Calcium needs to be given to the baby until its own body can take over. It is usually a result of prematurity.

- **Low magnesium:** This presents itself like low calcium and is also a result of prematurity.

- **Polycythaemia:** This condition, where too many red blood cells exist, occurs for unknown reasons. Blood is removed from the baby. The amount is determined by how much extra blood is present.

- **Respiratory distress syndrome:** This breathing problem occurs when the baby is delivered early, but it responds to treatment. It's rare with good prenatal care.

Your baby may be admitted to the special care nursery for observations if any of these complications are detected.

If the baby was exposed to high glucose and ketones during the pregnancy, it may show diminished intelligence. This is not obvious at birth but is discovered when the baby is expected to learn something.

The large baby of the poorly controlled mother with diabetes usually loses its fat within one year. Starting at ages six to eight, however, the child has a greater tendency to be obese. Controlling the blood glucose in the mother may prevent later obesity and even diabetes in the offspring.

Getting baby on the breast

Commencing breastfeeding as soon as possible after the birth is recommended because it provides essential nutrients and immune factors for the baby and also reduces the risk of low blood glucose levels in your baby. Holding your baby skin-to-skin (also known as *kangaroo care*) also keeps your baby warm and helps you bond with your new baby.

Establishing lactation can often begin prior to delivery. Nipple care and breast care during the antenatal period can help to ensure successful breastfeeding after your baby is born. Consult with your diabetes pregnancy care team or a lactation consultant for help with preparing for breastfeeding. Lactation consultants can also help with advice and support if you experience any problems with breastfeeding after the birth.

Large energy requirements are necessary during breastfeeding (just like other physical activity). If you have type 1 diabetes, it's important to check blood glucose levels before, during and after breastfeeding because blood glucose levels may drop.

 Have carbohydrate-containing food at hand to treat a rapid fall in blood glucose levels. Eating or drinking carbohydrate-containing foods such as a glass of milk, a slice of toast or a couple of plain biscuits while feeding can also reduce the risk of hypoglycaemia.

If you have type 1 diabetes, your insulin doses will need to be adjusted because breastfeeding women usually require less insulin.

 Although you are very busy after the birth of your baby, it's a good idea to touch base with your diabetes care team in the early weeks, when your food and insulin requirements are changing. They can assist you in looking after yourself!

For general information about caring for your baby after birth, and choosing the options that are best for baby and mother, see *Baby's First Year For Dummies*, Australian Edition, by Mara Lee (Wiley Publishing Australia Pty Ltd).

Checking for Diabetes After the Pregnancy

 If you had gestational diabetes, the diabetes usually disappears after delivery of the placenta. This is because the pregnancy hormones are lower and allow your own insulin to work more effectively in regulating blood glucose levels. However, a woman who develops gestational diabetes during pregnancy is at a much higher risk for later development of diabetes and obesity. Your baby is also at risk of developing childhood obesity and type 2 diabetes in later life.

If you had gestational diabetes, you need to have a 75-gram oral glucose tolerance test (OGTT) six to twelve weeks after pregnancy to check for diabetes. If diabetes is not found after the OGTT, you still need a fasting blood glucose level check annually (if you have a family history of type 2 diabetes) or every two years (if you have no family history).

Several factors predispose a woman with gestational diabetes to develop diabetes later on. Some factors can't be changed and include:

- **Age:** Pregnancies later in life triple the risk of permanent diabetes.
- **Ethnic origin:** Certain ethnic groups, such as Aboriginal Australians, Torres Strait Islanders, Asian Indians and Vietnamese, are at a higher risk.
- **Family history of diabetes:** If a family history is present, you are at a higher risk.
- **Number of pregnancies:** The more pregnancies you have, the higher your risk.
- **Pre-pregnancy weight:** Those with a higher pre-pregnancy weight are at a higher risk.
- **Severity of blood glucose during pregnancy:** Higher blood glucose levels mean a higher risk.

On the other hand, you can change or modify several factors:

- **Breastfeeding:** You and your baby will benefit if you are able to breastfeed.
- **Dietary fat:** Limit the fat in your diet, especially saturated fat.
- **Future pregnancies:** Have fewer children.
- **Future weight gain:** Gain less weight between pregnancies and during future pregnancies.
- **Physical activity:** Increase your activity to include 20 to 30 minutes of exercise, three to four times per week.
- **Smoking and certain drugs:** Stop smoking and using illicit drugs.

Women who have had gestational diabetes can use oral contraceptives with low levels of oestrogen and progesterone to prevent conception. These drugs, along with hormonal replacement therapy after menopause, don't increase your risk of later diabetes. Women with both type 1 and type 2 diabetes can use the same preparations.

Chapter 19

Occupational and Insurance Problems

. . . .

In This Chapter

▶ Finding work if you have diabetes

▶ Knowing the law is on your side

▶ Driving vehicles and flying planes

▶ Getting yourself health, travel and life insurance

. . . .

Most people need to work and some people even want to work. However, as a person with diabetes, you may come up against various forms of discrimination when you apply for a job. Part of it may be to do with fears for your health and safety if you work in remote locations, or fears that you may have a high number of sick days, which could affect your work output. Part of it has to do with a lack of understanding about diabetes and its management. Great strides have been made in diabetes care, so often a person with diabetes has a better work attendance record than a person without diabetes.

In this chapter, you find out what you need to know when you apply for work and various forms of insurance.

Employing People with Diabetes

In Australia, you should not be discriminated against in the workplace if you have diabetes. You only need to mention that you have diabetes if it's directly relevant to the duties that you carry out in your job, such as if the job requires you to work alone in isolated or dangerous locations (see the section 'Occupations with Restrictions' later in this chapter for more examples). But you must remember that if you don't tell your employer that you have diabetes, you may not be eligible to make workers compensation claims.

If diabetes is going to affect your work, show your employer that you're determined and flexible in making adjustments to your diabetic routine to suit your work environment. Make sure that you demonstrate a good understanding of diabetes and a responsible attitude towards your health.

When attending a job interview, take a letter of support from your doctor or endocrinologist outlining your diabetes profile and emphasising your commitment to your health.

Diabetes is not something that you should be ashamed about. Instead, emphasise the positive aspects that diabetes has had in the development of your healthy lifestyle.

In general, if your diabetes is controlled with diet or oral hypoglycaemic agents, you will experience fewer restrictions than if you are dependent on insulin to keep your blood glucose levels stable. Your employer may require you to have regular documented medical examinations and blood tests to monitor your diabetes status.

Diabetes can't be used as an excuse for not employing you unless strong evidence exists that having diabetes would genuinely prevent you from performing the duties outlined in your job specification (see also the following section). Assessment of any risks that may arise because you have diabetes is made on an individual basis.

Occupations with Restrictions

Occupational blanket bans on people with diabetes are rare, but certain occupations have restrictions in place to protect both you and your colleagues from dangerous situations. Examples of jobs that may put you and others at risk include the following:

- Commercial diving
- Commercial flying
- Long-distance truck driving and commercial bus driving
- Working alone in inaccessible or dangerous locations
- Working on offshore rigs

If a job requires unscheduled work for long periods of time without access to food or your medications, a real possibility exists of you becoming hypoglycaemic.

If you have diabetes, you may not be eligible to serve in the Australian Defence Force, because all defence force personnel should be able to be deployed to foreign countries where medical services may be poor or even non-existent. Each application is assessed on an individual basis. If you develop diabetes while you're in the defence force, depending on your role, your duties may need to be modified.

The police force also has a policy that doesn't encourage recruitment of people with diabetes. (Some cases of leniency can occur if diabetes is purely diet-controlled and seen to be stable.) If you develop diabetes while you are in the police force, your duties will probably be restricted to avoid situations such as high-speed chases, sieges and working in remote locations. These restrictions are determined after individual assessment.

The fire service individually assesses new recruits with diabetes to determine their level of blood glucose control.

Check with your local police and fire services as there may be some variation in individual state and territory policies.

The Law Is On Your Side

No discrimination laws deal specifically with diabetes but two laws cover possible discrimination as a consequence of having diabetes:

- ✔ The *Human Rights and Equal Opportunity Commission Act 1986*
- ✔ The *Disability Discrimination Act 1992*

Diabetes Australia acts as a consumer representative in discriminatory situations. If you feel that you've been treated unfairly directly as a result of having diabetes, contact your local branch, which will help you to determine your rights. Generally, cases are assessed individually, but as mentioned earlier, certain occupations and activities have restrictions in place for your protection and the safety of those around you.

Driving If You Have Diabetes

If you are diagnosed with diabetes and have a private car or motorcycle licence, you must by law notify the roads and transport authority in your state or territory and your insurance company immediately. If you're involved in an accident and have not informed both parties of your diabetes, you may not be covered.

If you are diet-controlled or are taking oral hypoglycaemic agents, you must get a medical review from your doctor and present a letter outlining the stability of your diabetes to the licensing department. The department will then decide how often you need to have a medical review. Generally, people who control their diabetes with diet don't require regular medical examination to maintain their licence. People who take oral hypoglycaemic agents usually require a medical examination every two to five years to maintain their licence, unless their diabetes is particularly unstable. People who are treated with insulin require a medical examination every one to two years to maintain their licence. Again, this is decided on an individual basis by your doctor in conjunction with the licensing authority.

If you are hospitalised for diabetic ketoacidosis or hypoglycaemia, your licence may be revoked until your condition is stable. Your fitness to return to driving will be up to your treating doctor to decide.

You can obtain a commercial licence for driving articulated or dangerous goods trucks, taxis or buses if your diabetes is diet-controlled or you are taking oral hypoglycaemic agents, as long as the licensing authority and your doctor agree, but each case is much more strictly and more frequently assessed than for private licences. Usually people with insulin-dependent diabetes are not eligible for this type of licence, but again it is at the discretion of the licensing authority and your doctor.

The National Health and Medical Research Council (NH&MRC) and the Australian Diabetes Society have developed an Australian policy on driving and diabetes in order to balance the rights and responsibilities of people with diabetes with the need to protect you and the general public from the consequences if you become hypoglycaemic while driving. The policy was heavily influenced by research that shows that diabetes is not a significant contributor to road accidents.

You must always be aware of the added responsibility of having diabetes and driving. It becomes even more important that you eat regularly, take your medications correctly and monitor your glucose levels. Make sure that you have with you at all times a source of sugar like jelly beans or glucose tablets and complex carbohydrate like fruit, dry biscuits or a sandwich. If you're intending to drive long distances, check your blood glucose before you drive and take regular meal breaks. If you develop any signs of hypoglycaemia, such as dizziness, shakiness, headache or loss of concentration, pull over to the side of the road immediately and turn off the engine. Then measure your blood glucose and treat with sugar or carbohydrate. Always wait until you have fully recovered before you start driving again.

Piloting a Plane

People with diabetes face restrictions on getting a pilot's licence. Although you can't obtain a commercial pilot's licence, the Civil Aviation Safety Authority (CASA) will individually assess people with diabetes who want to get a private pilot's licence. The assessment and review procedure is not as strict if you are diet-controlled or taking oral hypoglycaemic agents compared to if you are insulin-dependent. But don't lose heart if you require insulin: Your case will be considered. Getting a pilot's licence may not be easy but is well worth it for the person with diabetes who loves to fly.

For more information on applying for a licence to fly solo, go to the CASA website (`www.casa.gov.au`) and enter **insulin treated protocol** in the search option.

Obtaining Health Insurance

Choosing your health insurance policy is an important decision, particularly if you have diabetes. The correct choice can save you money in many areas of managing your condition. Each company has different schemes, so shop around and find the one that suits you best. The larger companies often have a standard pricing policy and a one-year waiting period for claims relating to all pre-existing conditions, including diabetes. However, each health insurance company has a different approach to this, depending on the type of cover you seek, so check this while you shop around.

Some of the areas where insurance companies provide rebates and discounts include

- ✔ Acupuncture
- ✔ Ambulance and hospital charges
- ✔ Glucose meters
- ✔ Insulin pumps
- ✔ Massage
- ✔ Medications
- ✔ Physiotherapy
- ✔ Visits to dietitians, endocrinologists and ophthalmologists

People with diabetes have the right to obtain health insurance at the same price rating as everyone else.

Obtaining Travel Insurance

Travel insurance is less regulated and you may well experience discrimination because of your diabetes when you apply to certain companies. Check whether your health insurance company offers additional travel insurance that will cover you if you require medical assistance while you are overseas.

Having insurance cover while travelling is essential, so if you're having trouble finding a company that will accept diabetes as an insurable condition, contact the Australian Diabetes Council (in NSW) or Diabetes Australia (in other states or territories). They are able to recommend insurance companies that are more understanding of your health status.

Obtaining Life Insurance

People with diabetes find that life insurance is the most difficult type of policy to obtain. When applying for life insurance, income protection insurance or recovery insurance you will often face loadings and exclusions. Diabetes is a difficult condition for insurance companies to consider because it's not a single disease — it can involve a whole group of complications including heart disease and renal disease. Shop around and find a company that will give you the best deal.

With life insurance, companies make a judgement by calculating your chance of dying and then either charge you an extra loading or turn you down based upon those calculations. This means the cost of life insurance is greater for people with diabetes than for those without it. Many companies use outdated statistics and calculations based on the life expectancy of people with diabetes determined years ago. Diabetes medicine has come a long way in a relatively short time. People who have diabetes are living a lot longer than they used to — make sure that the company you choose takes this into account.

As new studies are done, they should indicate that the life spans of people with and without diabetes are approaching equality. In some cases, people with diabetes take better care of themselves than people without a chronic illness and are living even longer. So the situation is improving and the insurance companies will catch up sooner or later. Can you imagine the surprise if insurance companies were ever to charge people with diabetes less than others because of their good habits?

Recovery insurance (offered by some companies) pays a lump sum if you develop one of 20 major illnesses. If you have diabetes, you're excluded from claiming for diabetes or diabetes-related illnesses like coronary artery disease and heart attack, kidney disease, retinopathy and neuropathy.

Your application for life insurance, income protection insurance or recovery insurance is based on a number of factors:

✔ An unbiased medical assessment of all aspects of your health

✔ Whether you smoke

✔ Your alcohol consumption

✔ Your blood pressure

✔ Your family history of disease

✔ Your weight

✔ Any additional lifestyle risks

From this, the extra loading that you're charged is calculated or a decision to reject your application is made. In most cases, the older you are when your diabetes is diagnosed, the more lenient the insurer will be as long as you haven't already developed other complications.

Chapter 20

Advances in Diabetes Care

*B*etween 1921, when insulin was isolated and used for the first time, and 1980, when blood glucose meters began to be available, relatively little was discovered about diabetes that improved diabetes care. Even in the years between 1980 and the mid-1990s, little progress was made. However, since 1995, the pace of discovery of new tests, new treatments and other products for diabetes has been remarkable.

While such drugs as metformin and sulphonylureas are established components of good diabetes care, many people now have access to new classes of oral medication (refer to Chapter 10). However, due to the increasingly heavy burden that diabetes places on the health care budget, doctors and researchers are aware of the urgent need to develop new therapies for diabetes. Many new developments have taken place overseas, particularly in the United States.

In this chapter, we cover treatments and medications for diabetes that may not be available in Australia yet but are available overseas. Before they can be released onto the Australian market, treatments must meet the strict and responsible standards laid down by the Therapeutic Goods Administration.

Note: We use the word *new* to describe treatments or medications that may come onto the Australian market in the near future and are therefore new at the date of publication of this book.

Monitoring Blood Glucose Levels

Although the devices currently available for monitoring blood glucose (refer to Chapter 9) are a great advance on earlier techniques, many still have their drawbacks: Testing may be painful and monitoring may be inconvenient — for example, certain people find monitoring difficult because of their physical disabilities.

One new device is aimed at making testing less painful. The Lasette laser lancing device, made by the American company Cell Robiotics International, uses a laser to puncture the skin. The Lasette works by burning a hole in the skin rather than by puncturing it with a needle.

Although some discomfort occurs with this device, the company claims that the discomfort doesn't last as long as that of a needle puncture. The device is quite expensive — the current model costs US$495 — and it's not currently approved for use in Australia.

Refer to Chapter 9 for more on continuous glucose monitoring devices that are more convenient and accurate, and now widely available in Australia.

Developing New Drugs and New Techniques

In the last few years, drug companies have made significant progress in producing drugs to alleviate the symptoms of both type 1 and type 2 diabetes. These companies have also focused on finding ways to deliver insulin without the need for injection. This section covers the drugs and techniques that show definite promise for people with diabetes.

Bringing new drugs onto the market

Advances in research have identified new targets in diabetes treatment. For example, hormones released from the gut have been found to be important in the control of blood glucose. Based on these findings, new drugs have become available and drugs that replace, mimic or improve the function of other hormones, not just insulin, are being sought.

A drug based on this new approach — exenatide (marketed as Byetta) — has emerged and is already in use. Exenatide is an injection given two times per day before breakfast and dinner — very similar to how insulin is given. The medication mimics the natural gut hormone *glucagon-like peptide-1* (GLP-1), which lowers glucose levels after a meal by stimulating insulin release. Exenatide has the advantage over insulin of not causing hypoglycaemia (unless it's combined with another diabetes medication known to lower glucose) and it may cause some weight loss. The main side effect is nausea.

In patients who don't wish to have injections, an alternative is sitagliptin (marketed as Januvia), or vildagliptin (marketed as Galvus), which can be taken orally. These medications prevent the breakdown of GLP-1.

Another promising target is a synthetic version of *amylin*, a hormone in the pancreas that's secreted with insulin in response to food intake. Research has shown that amylin also helps regulate glucose levels.

Amylin therapy as an adjunct to treatment with insulin may be an important therapeutic option for improving glucose control in patients with type 1 diabetes and in people with type 2 diabetes who are on insulin. However, like insulin, amylin is administered via a subcutaneous injection. It's not currently available for use in Australia.

Improving insulin delivery

Whenever people hear that they need to be on insulin, the most common reaction — and biggest hurdle they have to overcome — is the fear of having multiple injections. As a result of this fear, drug companies are working on ways to deliver insulin without needles. This section sets out the latest developments in insulin delivery; many of the new ways to deliver insulin may come on to the market in the near future.

Oral insulin

The difficulty with taking insulin by mouth is that it is a large protein and proteins are broken down by digestive enzymes into individual amino acids. So, in order to effectively take insulin by mouth, you need a device to protect the insulin from those digestive enzymes.

One way that insulin can be taken orally is to package the insulin in 'biologically erodable microspheres'. These tiny round packages can carry insulin through the intestinal lining, where it's released in an active form into the blood stream. The packages later break up and leave the body.

The developmental work on oral insulin is in the early stages and such a drug is a long way from being released onto the market. However, oral insulin is something you should know about, because you may be taking insulin this way in the future.

Inhaled insulin

An inhaled form of insulin was available for a short time in Australia, offering the first new insulin delivery option since insulin's discovery in the 1920s. Studies showed that inhaled insulin (marketing as Exubera) was just as effective as injected insulin in its ability to control the blood glucose in both type 1 and type 2 diabetes. However, Exubera was discontinued at the end of 2007 because of lower than expected sales. The low sales were probably related to inconvenience and side effects such as a sore throat and dry cough.

A different inhaled insulin preparation, which appears to have greater dosing flexibility and a more convenient delivery system, is in clinical trials.

Transdermal insulin

Another mode of insulin delivery being explored is *transdermal delivery*, where the medication is delivered through the skin. This is a convenient method, and has been used for the delivery of several hormones in the treatment of hormonal disorders. For example, transdermal oestrogen delivery, in the form of skin patches, has been used for a long time in hormone therapy for women.

The biggest challenge in transdermal delivery is the passage of the medication through the outermost layer of skin. Insulin, being a relatively big molecule, can't pass through this outer layer. Research has, therefore, focused on the use of *microneedle technology*. This involves a 'poke-and-patch' device, where microneedles on a patch pierce the skin to allow insulin to be delivered to the fatty layer underneath the skin. Because the needles on the patch are so small, spontaneous healing of the skin occurs after the patch has been applied.

Transdermal insulin has shown some success in animal studies. Whether it's as effective in humans, and whether enough people prefer a patch with microneedles to a relatively painless insulin pen, awaits further research.

Implantable insulin

A delivery method also being researched is the implantable insulin pump, which is implanted under the skin and delivers insulin either to the abdominal cavity or directly to the liver. Like the external insulin pumps already available (refer to Chapter 10), the implantable pump delivers background insulin as well as food-related insulin. It is a disc-shaped device weighing between 180 and 240 grams.

Studies of about 70 patients have shown that the pump can successfully deliver insulin for up to four years or even longer. The patients in the studies had good metabolic control without a lot of weight gain. However, problems have occurred with infection at the implantation site, necessitating removal of the pump.

This method of insulin delivery is still very much in the experimental stage and is currently unavailable in Australia.

Transplanting the Pancreas or Insulin-producing Cells

If you have type 1 diabetes, all you need is a new pancreas — and you're cured. If only it were that simple! The problem, of course, is that your body doesn't like to have someone else's pancreas inside it, and it tends to reject the foreign tissue and destroy it.

The only way to protect a transplanted organ is to block the body's rejection mechanism, called the *immune response*. Several drugs can block the immune response, but in so doing, they create problems of their own. For example, corticosteroids may block the immune response but they also have the effect of raising blood glucose.

One treatment for kidney failure is transplantation of a new kidney (refer to Chapter 7). Until effective treatments are available to prevent rejection of pancreatic cells, transplants of the pancreas are usually only considered when a person with diabetes is undergoing a life-saving kidney transplant. Pancreas transplantations have many benefits:

✔ Patients suffering from hypoglycaemia, hyperglycaemia or autonomic problems (refer to Chapter 7) have an improved quality of life.

✔ Progression of complications already present may be slowed or stopped.

✔ The new kidney is exposed to normal blood glucose levels.

The choice of the recipient of the transplant is important because certain factors influence success:

✔ Being over 45 years of age can result in a less positive prognosis.

✔ Congestive heart failure results in a poor prognosis.

✔ Hardening of the arteries already present is a negative factor.

✔ Hepatitis C infection increases the risk of transplant loss.

✔ Obesity also increases the risk of transplant loss.

Due to the high incidence of post-operative illness associated with pancreas transplantation, as well as a lifelong requirement for immunosuppression, a simultaneous kidney and pancreas transplantation is, therefore, only a definite option for a younger person with type 1 diabetes who has kidney failure and needs a transplant. Such people would receive a new kidney at the same time as they receive a new pancreas.

Data from the transplant unit at a major teaching hospital have shown that more than 80 per cent of patients who get a new pancreas no longer need insulin and maintain normal glucose levels after the operation. However, if the side effects of pancreas transplantation surgery could be minimised, or immunosuppression improved, then this treatment could be made available to a larger number of patients.

Another approach is to transplant the insulin-producing tissue (islet cells) into the liver. Islets are taken from the pancreas of a deceased organ donor. The islets are purified, processed, and transferred into the person with type 1 diabetes. Soon after implantation these islets begin to make and release insulin. However, full islet function and new blood vessel growth associated with the islets takes time and insulin is given until the islets are fully functional. With this method, lifelong immunosuppression is still required.

So far, transplanting islet cells has only been moderately successful. A proportion of patients have been able to come off insulin injections, and the insulin-producing cells of even fewer patients continue to function one year after the operation. One of the reasons for this is that, although the cells continue to work and make insulin, they are attacked by the immune system and become covered with a layer of other cells, in a process called *fibrosis*. The result is that the blood glucose can't get in to trigger the production of insulin and its release, and the insulin can't get out.

Some researchers are currently working on a technique called *microencapsulation*, which involves covering these insulin-producing cells with thin membranes that protect these cells from immune attack while still allowing insulin to get into the blood stream. This may reduce the need for immunosuppressant drugs (and their unwanted side effects).

New studies are also focusing on identifying islet-producing stem cells and experimental ways to 'grow' islets. For example, some preliminary success suggests that stem cells from human embryos can be stimulated to become insulin-producing cells. Other researchers are working on purifying islets cultured from animals, such as pigs, which may be another source of cells capable of making insulin.

Chapter 21

What Doesn't Work When You're Treating Diabetes

*E*veryone wants a quick and easy solution to their problems. For every problem, five people offer a quick and easy answer. Just send in the money. These cheats have got what it takes to take what you've got.

The purpose of this chapter is to tell you as much as we know about the tests and treatments that don't work. Don't expect to find everything you have heard or read about that is 'the new wonder cure' for diabetes. As soon as this book is published, new, more seductive claims will be made. We hope that you will remain sceptical, use the information, especially in the first section, to test them out, and check with your GP or diabetes care team before you stop what works and try something that may do more harm than good.

If you're about to try a new therapy that has not been recommended by your GP and it is not discussed in this book, you may want to contact the Australian Diabetes Society or Diabetes Australia to find out their position on the treatment. Of course, if you're involved in a clinical trial that is trying to determine the effectiveness of a treatment, no-one will know whether it works or not.

Finding What Will Work for You

Many clues can alert you to the fact that a treatment may not work. Here are some of them:

- **If a treatment is endorsed by a Hollywood star or a football player or other sports figure, be highly sceptical.** Always consider the source and make sure that it's reputable. In this case, it's the fame of the star that is being used to convince you, not any special knowledge that he or she possesses.

- **If the treatment has been around for a long time but is not generally used, don't trust it.** Treatments that really work will have been tried in an experimental study where some people take it and some don't. Doctors and medical texts recommend drugs that pass that test.

- **If it sounds too good to be true, it usually is.** An example would be the claims about any products that say you don't have to change your diet or increase your exercise to lose weight.

- **Anecdotes are not proof of the value of a treatment or test.** The favourable experiences of one or a few people are not a substitute for a scientific study. If they did seem to respond to the drug, it may be for entirely different reasons.

A lot of the information is available on the internet. In Chapter 24, we provide several web addresses of the best resources currently available for diabetes. When you consider the validity of claims made on the Web, bear in mind the hints about detecting dodgy claims that we gave you earlier in this section and also note the following:

- **Don't rely on search engines.** Search engines do not check claims of validity.

- **Go to the site of the claim and check to see whether most of the information there makes sense.** A lot of silly information should alert you. If you still feel the treatment might work, ask the webmaster for references. If none are forthcoming, forget about the idea.

- **Go to sites that you know are reliable to see whether you can find the same recommendations.** The treatments on sites like Diabetes Australia, the Australian Diabetes Society and the International Diabetes Federation can be relied upon. When there is uncertainty, these sites can usually tell you.

Check which type of diabetes the information is relevant to, because significant differences exist between the types of diabetes and thus the treatments and information required. In general, the majority of the commonly found information (particularly that promoted in the media) relates to type 2 diabetes, unless it specifies otherwise.

Your health and the internet

The Health on the Net Foundation has established a set of principles that any site on the internet can adhere to. A site that follows the HONcode principles has agreed to the following principles:

Principle 1: Medical advice will be given by qualified professionals, or it will be stated that this is not the case.

Principle 2: The information supports but does not replace the patient–doctor relationship.

Principle 3: Confidentiality of visitors to the site is respected.

Principle 4: Information on the site is supported by references and dates.

Principle 5: Claims about the benefit of specific treatments are supported by references.

Principle 6: Information is provided in the clearest possible manner with contacts provided for more information, including the webmaster's email address.

Principle 7: Support for the site is clearly identified, especially commercial support.

Principle 8: If supported by advertising, it is clearly stated, along with the advertising policy. Advertising is clearly differentiated from non-advertising material.

If a site agrees with these principles, you can bet the information on it is very reliable.

Staying Clear of the Shonky Stuff

In the last decade, so many drugs have been touted as the cure for diabetes, you would think everyone would be cured by now. The fact is, as we have said again and again, you do have the tools right now to control diabetes, but it is not as simple as taking a tablet. If it were, this book would not be necessary. In this section, we tell you about some drugs that have usually become well known because they 'worked' in a few people.

A system is in place to protect you in the form of clinical research trials. Make sure that your trial has been approved by an ethics committee or review board in an institution that has been approved to do the research.

Dosing on chromium

In all kinds of magazines and on the internet, you can find articles singing the praises of chromium for its ability to control the symptoms of diabetes. Should you take supplements of chromium?

The strongest case for chromium comes from a study of people in China with type 2 diabetes. They were given high doses of chromium and were found to improve their glycosylated HbA1c, blood glucose and cholesterol while reducing the amount of insulin they had to take. However, these people were found to be chromium deficient in the first place. People in Australia and other countries where the diet provides adequate chromium don't show chromium deficiency and don't show improvement in glucose tolerance when they take chromium. In addition, chromium is present in such small amounts normally that it's hard to measure even in people without chromium deficiency. Chromium has never been shown to be of benefit to those with type 1 diabetes.

The amount of chromium that a person needs in their diet is uncertain but is estimated to be between 25 and 35 micrograms daily. People given much more than that tend to accumulate it in their liver, where it can be toxic. Some studies suggest that chromium can cause cancer in high doses.

For now, the answer is that the evidence does not support the use of chromium in diabetes except where the person is known to be chromium deficient.

Being careful with aspirin

People who take the sulphonylurea drugs (refer to Chapter 10) sometimes have a greater drop in blood glucose when they take aspirin. This is because aspirin competes with the other drug for binding sites on the proteins that carry sulphonylureas in the blood. When they're bound to protein, the sulphonylureas are not active but when they're free, they are. Aspirin knocks the sulphonylureas off so that they're free. As a result, aspirin has been recommended as a drug to lower blood glucose.

By itself, aspirin has little effect on blood glucose. Its effect with sulphonylureas is so inconsistent that it can't be reliably depended upon to lower the blood glucose.

What about hypnosis?

Some sources recommend hypnosis as a treatment for the 'stabilisation of blood sugar in diabetes'. No experimental evidence exists that proves the usefulness of hypnosis. So you have to be wary of this and other areas of alternative or complementary medicine that might claim to be able to control blood glucose levels.

Rejecting pancreas formula

Pancreas formula is sold on the internet as a mixture of herbs, vitamins and minerals that help diabetes. No clinical or experimental evidence shows that pancreas formula does anything of value in the human body. The claims that are made for this 'treatment' are not supported by factual evidence. Look for references in respected journals, and you will not find them. Save your money.

Giving FatBlaster a miss

You will have seen a lot of advertising for the FatBlaster products on television and on the internet. Advertisements claim that you can 'burn fat without diet or exercise'. This is equivalent to waving a magic wand. In order to burn fat, you need to exercise more and stop consuming large amounts of kilojoules. The products from this company include FatBlaster Fat Absorber, FatBlaster Fat Magnet, and FatBlaster tablets. No scientific evidence exists to prove that any of these products work! Their claims are based on rather crazy theories about how your body works.

Many weight loss products similar to FatBlaster can be found in pharmacies and on the internet — this book isn't long enough to list them all! Always check with your GP before taking any such products and know that if your GP isn't prescribing them it's because they don't work!

Accepting aspartame

You may come across a claim in the media that aspartame causes cancer. Because aspartame is used so much by people with and without diabetes, we want to emphasise the following.

Aspartame is an acceptable artificial sweetener with no known dangers to human beings. No evidence shows that aspartame causes cancer when used in normal amounts. It is inconceivable that anyone would use more than the recommended average daily intake (which includes a large safety factor). Food Standards Australia New Zealand does not support the view that it is carcinogenic — otherwise, it would have been withdrawn from use.

Recognising the Diets that Don't Work

If you walk into a reasonably large bookshop, you will be overwhelmed by the number of diet books. It may be a fair statement that the more books that are written about a subject, the less that is known for certain about that subject. Why would authors bother to come up with ten new books on dieting each year, if the solution rested in some older book? You can bet that word of mouth would have made that book the all-time bestseller in any category.

The books are way too numerous to list here by name, but they can be broken down into a few categories:

- **Diets that promote a lot of protein with little carbohydrate:** The trouble with these diets is that they're not a healthy and balanced approach. Unless you use tofu as your source of protein, you will be getting a lot of fat in your diet, much of it saturated fat. That is not good for you. The diet is lacking in vitamins that a supplemental vitamin tablet may or may not provide. Very few people stay on such a diet for long. How many people can eat chicken for breakfast, lunch and dinner? The diet is also lacking in potassium, an essential mineral.

  People who do follow this kind of diet for a long time also find that they have problems with hair loss, cracking nails and dry skin. Their breath and their urine smell of acetone because of all the fat breakdown. They become very dry and need to drink large quantities of fluid.

  We see a place for this diet as a starter. Some people with type 2 diabetes who have high blood glucose levels show rapid improvement when started on a diet like this. As the glucose comes under control, the diet can be changed to a more balanced one.

- **Diets that promote little or no fat:** The people who can follow a diet that is less than 20 per cent fat deserve a new designation — fatnatics (fat fanatics). This kind of diet is extremely difficult to prepare and perhaps even more difficult to eat unless you're a rabbit. In order to make up the kilojoules, people on this diet eat large amounts of carbohydrate. Chapter 11 makes it clear why this is not a good idea for people with diabetes.

  Like the protein diet, this diet may be lacking in essential vitamins and minerals, especially the fat-soluble vitamins. It, too, may be a good way to start a dietary program for a person with type 2 diabetes, as long as the total kilojoules are not greater than the daily needs of that individual.

✓ **Very low kilojoule diets:** Many versions of these diets are currently on the market. These diets are often in the form of a liquid meal replacement, which contains kilojoules but may not taste very good. Some of these diets are lacking in many essential nutrients and they must be supplemented by vitamins and minerals. Others are complete and don't require additional supplementation. They can't form the basis of a permanent diet because eventually everyone must go back to eating proper food. They are designed to be taken continuously for three to six months and then food is gradually reintroduced. The key to success is putting back *less* food than you were originally taking in! If you go back to your old diet, you will put all the weight back on — and sometimes more. Another important element in the long-term success of this approach is increasing your level of physical activity — this helps you to reduce the regain of weight that comes after these diets have finished.

Not all doctors or dietitians like this kind of diet even as a starter diet because it is so unlike our usual eating habits that some people rapidly find it to be intolerable. Eating is a basic part of human existence. Eating can be done alone, but it's more enjoyable in company. It's a source of great pleasure for human beings and other animals. A diet that takes away this fundamental activity will not be tolerated for very long. This is why they should be seen as a relatively short-term intervention and expert advice from a dietitian should be sought before going on one of these programs.

The transition from a very low kilojoule diet to a balanced diet is a very difficult one. Success depends on getting help from your diabetes care team to support you through the process.

For the overweight person with type 2 diabetes, any diet that results in some weight loss helps for a time. But you have to ask yourself the following questions:

✓ Am I prepared to stay on this diet indefinitely?

✓ Is it a diet that is healthy if I stay on it?

✓ Will it combine all the features I need — weight loss, reduction of blood glucose and reduction of blood fat levels — with palatability and reasonable cost?

If you can say yes to all those questions, then the diet will probably work for you.

Rapid weight loss will also require a rapid adjustment of medication — both for your blood glucose and blood pressure. Keep in touch with your diabetes care team to make sure this happens appropriately.

Part VI
The Part of Tens

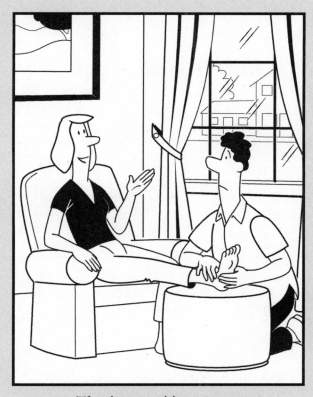

'The doctor told me it was crucial that 1 receive hour-long foot massages every day.'

In this part . . .

In this part, you get key techniques for managing diabetes. With just a little background from the other parts, you can use these chapters to really finetune your diabetes care. You also get the ten commandments of excellent care, along with ten major myths about diabetes that you can discard. Finally, we cut through the enormous amount of information available online to give you the best — and most reliable — websites to access for more help with your diabetes management.

Chapter 22

Ten Ways to Prevent or Reverse the Effects of Diabetes

*1*f you have read everything that came before this, congratulations. But we didn't expect you to (and besides, this is a reference book, not a novel) and that's why we wrote this chapter. Follow the leaders' (our) advice in this chapter, and you can be in great shape with your diabetes.

Monitoring Your Blood Glucose

You have your glucose meter. Now what do you do with it? Most people do not like to prick themselves and are reluctant to do so at first. How often you test is between you and your doctor, but the more you do it, the easier it will be to control your diabetes. Monitoring gives you more insight into your particular response to food, exercise and medications. (Refer to Chapter 9 for more on monitoring blood glucose.)

People with type 1 diabetes need to test before meals and at bedtime because their blood glucose level determines their dose of insulin. Sometimes your diabetes care team may also ask you to test one or two hours after a meal or overnight in special circumstances (such as pregnancy). This gives your team further information to help you to get your blood glucose levels where you want them to be.

People who have stable type 2 diabetes may test once per day at different times or more often if medication is changing or if readings seem higher than usual.

Always take your blood glucose readings along when visiting your GP or any of the members of your diabetes care team — the more information everyone has about you, the more specific the advice and assistance provided.

If you're sick or about to start a long drive, you might want to test more often because you don't want to become hypoglycaemic — or hyperglycaemic for that matter. The beauty of the meter is that you can check your blood glucose in less than 30 seconds any time you feel it's necessary.

Being Careful with What You Eat

If you are what you eat, you have a pretty good incentive to consider your consumption carefully. If you gain weight, you gain insulin resistance, but it doesn't take a lot of weight loss to reverse the situation. The main point you should understand about a diet for diabetes is that it's a healthy diet for anyone, whether they have diabetes or not. You shouldn't feel like a social outcast because you're eating the right foods. You don't need special supplements; the diet is balanced and contains all the vitamins and minerals you require (although you want to be sure you're getting enough calcium).

If you think your diet may be unbalanced, consult your GP or see your diabetes dietitian for a full nutritional assessment.

You can follow a diet for diabetes wherever you are, not just at home. Every menu has something on it that's appropriate for you. If you're invited to someone's home, tell your host you have diabetes and to be unconcerned if you don't accept the offer of seconds or a large portion of dessert! Sometimes strictly controlling the amount of fat or carbohydrate that you eat, or your portion size, is not possible, so you need to accept the fact that your diet will not always be perfect and go on from there. (Refer to Chapter 11 for more on your diet.)

Having Tests Regularly

The people who make smoke detectors recommend that you change the battery without fail each time the clocks go back at the end of daylight saving. If you live in a state or territory without daylight saving, you need to use another regular event, such as your birthday. You should use the same simple device to remember your 'complication detectors'. Make sure that your doctor checks your urine for tiny amounts of protein and your feet for loss of sensation every year. Once you know the problem is present, you can do a lot to slow it down or even reverse it. Never has it been more true that 'an ounce of prevention is worth a pound of cure'. (For more on complications you may develop, refer to Chapters 6 and 7.)

We've made it very easy for you to know about the tests you need at the time you need them — the testing recommendations are all in Chapter 7. Be insistent that you get the tests when they are due. A GP with a busy medical practice may forget whether you have had the tests you need, but if you have a reminder system for yourself, you will be less likely to forget.

Keeping Active

Keeping active can help your diabetes in many different ways. It can help your muscles become more sensitive to insulin, it may help you lose weight and it can reduce your risk of heart disease. Exercise can be used to burn up glucose in place of insulin, thereby lowering your blood glucose even without losing weight.

Those with type 1 diabetes need to adjust their insulin around their physical activity — for help with this, refer to Chapter 12 and check with your diabetes care team. It might take a little more effort to work out your new insulin requirements once you start exercising, but it's worth it because of all the great benefits exercise can bring to your life.

We're not talking about an hour of running or 100 kilometres on the bike. Moderate exercise like brisk walking can accomplish the same thing. The key is to exercise regularly. (For more on exercise, refer to Chapter 12.)

Educating Yourself

When we see a patient new to us who has been diagnosed with diabetes for some time, it's often amazing to find that this poor person has not been given any education about the fundamentals of diabetes. How can you live more comfortably and avoid complications if someone doesn't help you to learn all that's required to care for your diabetes?

So much is going on in the field of diabetes that even we have trouble keeping up with it, and it's our speciality! How can you expect to know when the doctors come up with the major advances that will cure your diabetes? The answer is lifelong learning.

Once you have got past the shock of the diagnosis, you're ready to learn. This book contains a lot of basic information that you need to know. You can even take a course in diabetes self-management. These are often provided by local diabetes care teams or in community health centres. The Australian Diabetes Council (in NSW) or Diabetes Australia (in other states and territories) also run courses and can help you find the closest ones to you.

Then you need to keep learning. Become a member of Diabetes Australia and get access to the terrific magazine called *Conquest,* which usually contains information on the state of the art in diabetes management. In some states the publication may not be directly posted to you. If you go to the Diabetes Australia website (see Chapter 24) you can access past copies online. Diabetes Australia is also working with Pacific Magazines to provide editorial review of their magazine *Diabetic Living,* which is available in newsagencies and supermarkets.

Of course, you can also go to the websites that we discuss in Chapter 24 for a wide range of suggested and reputable information.

Remember that a lot of misinformation is available on the Web, so you must be careful to check out a recommendation before you start to follow it (refer to Chapter 21). Even information on reliable sites may not be right for your particular problem.

Heeding the Doctor's Advice

Treating your disease in accordance with your doctor's instructions is always beneficial. Certainly, it's a pain (even if you could take insulin by mouth and not by injection). The basic assumption in diabetes care is that you're taking your medication regularly — your doctor bases all his or her decisions on that assumption. Some very serious mistakes can be made if that assumption is false. Diabetes medications are pretty potent, and too much of a good thing can be bad for you. (For more on medications, refer to Chapter 10.)

Every time a study is done on why people with diabetes don't do better, the lack of regularity in taking medications is high up or leads the list of reasons. Do you make a conscious decision to miss your tablets, or do you forget? Perhaps just not enough money is left at the end of the month for the script to be filled. Whatever the reason, the best thing to do is to set up a system that helps you to remember. Keeping your tablets in a dated container quickly shows you if you have taken them or not. You might even divide the tablets by time of day. Make the system simple so that it will work for you. Speak with your diabetes care team if finances are a problem — they may be able to help.

Maintaining a Positive Outlook

Your approach to your condition can go a long way towards determining whether you live in diabetes heaven or diabetes hell. It can help to see your diabetes as a challenge and an opportunity.

Diabetes is a challenge because you have to think about doing certain things that others never have to worry about. It brings out the quality of organisation, which can then be transferred to other parts of your life.

Diabetes is an opportunity because it encourages you to make healthy choices for your diet as well as your exercise. You may well end up a lot healthier than your neighbour without diabetes. As you make more and more healthy choices, you feel and test less and less like a person with diabetes. Does this mean that at some point you can give up your treatment? Probably not, although you will most likely be able to take less medication — and you will feel a lot better!

Does diabetes mean that you can't do what you want to do in your life? The person with diabetes has only a few legal restrictions, and they're disappearing fast. (Refer to Chapter 19 for more on this.) Diabetes doesn't need to stop you having a full and enjoyable life.

Refer to Chapter 13 for lots of good advice on how to get your positive feelings going.

Being Prepared

Life is full of surprises. You never know when you will get more than you bargained for. That's why having a plan to deal with the unexpected is useful.

You run into great stress at work or at home. Does this throw you off your diet, your exercise and taking your medications? You go off travelling and get food poisoning or an upset stomach. Are you prepared and do you know what to do?

The key to these situations is the realisation that it's not possible for everything to go right all the time. You must be prepared for the times when things go wrong. This book is all about 'what to do if'. The more you understand the information available in this book, the less often you will find yourself in a situation that you can't handle.

You might even do a 'dry run'. Go to the website of a restaurant that you might like to try and read their menu. Think about and select the foods that will help you to stay in control. If you have questions, ask your diabetes care team. Practising handling these situations before they arise makes it a lot easier to function when you are faced with the real thing.

Examining Your Feet

A recent headline read: 'Hospital sued by seven foot doctors'. We would certainly not like to treat any doctor with seven feet or even a doctor who is seven feet tall. Whether you have two feet or seven feet, you must take good care of them.

Although diabetes is a major source of foot amputations, these kinds of operations are entirely preventable — but you must pay attention to your feet. Problems occur when you can't feel with your feet because of neuropathy (refer to Chapter 7). You can easily find out when this is present by getting your GP to check with a monofilament. If your feet can't feel the filament, they may not feel burning hot water, a stone or nail in your shoe or an infected ulcer on your foot.

Once you lose sensation in your feet, your eyes must replace the pain fibres that would otherwise tell you a problem is developing. You need to examine your feet carefully every day, keep your toenails trimmed and wear comfortable shoes. Your GP should be inspecting your feet at every visit.

Test bath water by hand, shake your shoes out before you put them on and wear new shoes only for a short while before checking for pressure spots. The future of your feet is in your hands. (Refer to Chapter 8 for more on caring for your feet.)

Focusing On Your Eyes

You're reading this book, which means you're seeing this book. So far, there are no plans to put out a braille edition, so you better take care of your eyes or you will miss out on the wonderful gems of information that brighten every page.

Eyecare starts with a careful examination by an optometrist or ophthalmologist. You need to have an exam at least once per year (or more often if necessary). If your diabetes is well controlled, the doctor will find two normal eyes. If not, signs of diabetic eye disease may show up (refer to Chapter 7). At that point, you need to control your diabetes, which means controlling your blood glucose. You also want to control your blood pressure because high blood pressure contributes to worsening eye disease.

Although the final word is not in on the effects of smoking and excessive alcohol on eye disease in diabetes, is it worth risking your sight for another puff of a cigarette? Even at this late stage, you can stop the progression of the eye disease or reverse some of the damage.

Chapter 23

Ten Myths about Diabetes That You Can Forget

In This Chapter

▶ Doing exactly the right thing yields a perfect glucose every time

▶ Giving into temptation can kill you

▶ And more myths you shouldn't believe

*M*yths are a lot of fun. They're never completely true, but you can usually find a tiny bit of truth in a myth — which is one reason (along with the need for an explanation when 'science' fails to provide one) so many myths are believed.

The trouble is that some myths can harm you if you allow them to determine your medical care. This chapter is about those kinds of myths — the ones that lead you to not take your medication or eat a well-balanced diet or even to take things that may not be good for you. The ten myths in this chapter are only a small sample of all the myths that exist about diabetes. They could take up a whole book on their own. But the myths we describe here are some of the more important ones. Realising that these are myths can help prevent you from making some serious mistakes about good diabetes care.

Following Treatment Perfectly Yields Perfect Glucose Levels

Doctors are probably as responsible as their patients are for the myth that perfect treatment results in perfect glucoses. For decades, doctors measured the urine glucose and told their patients that if they would just stay on their diet, take their medication and get their exercise, the urine would be negative for glucose.

Doctors failed to account for the many variables that could result in a positive test for glucose in the urine, plus the fact that even if the urine was negative, the patient could still be experiencing diabetic damage (because the urine becomes negative at a blood glucose of around 10 mmol/L in most people, a level that still causes damage).

The same thing is true for the blood glucose. Although you can achieve normal blood glucose levels most of the time if you treat your diabetes properly, you can still have times when, for no apparent reason, the glucose is not normal. When you consider that so many factors can determine the blood glucose level at any given time, this variation should hardly be a surprise. These factors include:

✔ Your diet

✔ Your exercise

✔ Your medication

✔ Your emotional state

✔ Other illnesses

✔ The day of your menstrual cycle (if a woman)

The miracle is that the blood glucose is what you expect it to be as often as it is. Don't allow an occasional unexpected result to throw you. Keep on doing what you know to be right, and your overall control will be excellent.

Eating a Slice of Cake Can Kill You

Some people can become fanatical when they develop diabetes. They think that they must be perfect in every aspect of their diabetes care and can drive themselves crazy with their belief that they must always follow the 'perfect diet' all the time.

Now, doctors may be at fault here, having told their patients that they must avoid sugar at all costs! As Chapter 11 shows, doctors and your diabetes care team now understand that a little sugar in the diet is not harmful. They also appreciate that some regular 'treat' foods can be helpful in keeping you motivated to keep eating well for the majority of the time.

This myth goes back again to the fact that science doesn't have all the answers. Knowledge is still evolving. It may never reach the point where the statement made to Woody Allen's character in the movie *Sleeper* is true. He wakes up after sleeping for 100 years and is told that scientists now realise that milkshakes and fatty meats are good for you. But who knows?

The bottom line is occasional dietary lapses aren't harmful. No-one is perfect — not even your diabetes care team, and not even you! Don't feel the need to have a perfect diet all the time.

You Can Tell the Level of Your Blood Glucose by How You Feel

Actually, this is a very common myth that people tell us all the time. To look at this scientifically, a research study was conducted whereby people with diabetes were hooked up to glucose and insulin intravenous lines so researchers could manipulate their blood glucose levels.

Participants were 'given' a particular blood glucose level and asked to say what it was. The number of correct answers was pretty bad — most people couldn't even accurately tell if they were hypoglycaemic (blood glucose too low) or hyperglycaemic (blood glucose too high)!

The moral of the story: Test your blood glucose at your required intervals, and especially if you think you are high or low. Guessing may lead you in exactly the wrong direction with your treatment, which will cause more problems.

Finding a Cure in Unorthodox Methods

In Chapter 21, we talk about some treatments that don't work. Those treatments were just the tip of the iceberg. Many treatments will not help you and may harm you. Whenever a problem affects a huge number of people, others are eager to exploit this potential goldmine.

How can you know if what you read in your favourite magazine or see on the internet is actually useful? Check it out with your GP, your diabetes educator or other members of your diabetes care team (refer to Chapter 14). They will know or can find out for you about any appropriate treatment. To date, diabetes has no simple cures. A book or organisation that promises an easy cure is not doing you any favours.

Diabetes Ends Spontaneity

You may think that your freedom to eat when you want and come and go as you please is gone once you have diabetes. This myth is far from the truth. If you have type 1 diabetes, you need to balance your insulin intake with your food intake, but the availability of newer insulins means you can eat just about when you want and take your rapid-acting insulin (refer to Chapter 10) just before or even during or right after you eat. If you're a heavy exerciser, even the need for much insulin may not be true. A very small number of type 1 patients take only a few units of insulin because they are so physically active.

Do you have to give up eating out if you have diabetes? Of course not — it's one of life's great pleasures! Newer oral agents for type 2 diabetes allow you to eat when you want and anticipate that the blood glucose levels will remain within or close to target range.

Should you dance the night away even though you have diabetes? Of course you should! Cut back on your insulin because you'll be doing more exercise and check your blood glucose once or twice during the night. Other than that, go for it! Naturally, exercise helps the type 2 patient as well, and oral medications are unlikely to need adjustment for these occasional situations.

Can you travel where you want with diabetes? Most certainly. You just need to plan your trip in advance so you can get together all the bits and pieces you need in time. For example, make sure that you have a list of your medications with you to show customs if requested. Keep your medications with you so that if your luggage gets lost, your medicine doesn't go with it. Purchase travel insurance (refer to Chapter 19) — even if it's a bit more expensive because of your diabetes, it's invaluable if you have the misfortune of something going wrong while you're overseas. These three things are now simple to do and ensure that diabetes will not affect your trip.

Needing Insulin Means You're Doomed

Many people with type 2 diabetes believe that once they have to take insulin, they're on a rapid downhill course to death. This is not true. Once you're using insulin, it probably means that your pancreas has conked out and can't produce enough insulin to control your blood glucose, even when stimulated by oral drugs. But taking insulin is no more a death sentence for you than it is for the person with type 1 diabetes.

Sometimes using insulin is a temporary measure for when you're very sick with some other illness that makes your oral drugs ineffective. Once the illness is over, your need for insulin ends.

Other times, insulin is commenced because the oral medications you're using can no longer keep your blood glucose levels in the target range and using insulin is your only alternative to keep you well.

The majority of people with type 2 diabetes eventually end up needing insulin injections. If the recent jump in the number of new medications used to manage diabetes is any indication of things to come, this may soon become a thing of the past; however, for now, if you do require insulin try not to be afraid or anxious about it. Your diabetes care team are there to help you cope with a new way to manage your diabetes and will make the process as easy for you as possible.

Occasionally people with diabetes who have been on insulin for some time after 'failing' oral agents can be taken off the insulin and given one of the newer oral agents, which actually controls their glucose better than the insulin. One typical patient was on 40 units of insulin weighing 82 kilograms with an HbA1c of 7.4 per cent. His insulin dose was gradually lowered as Byetta (refer to Chapter 10) was added to his treatment. He lost 5 kilograms, came off insulin entirely and now has a HbA1c of 6.5 per cent.

Older people with diabetes may need insulin to keep their blood glucose at a reasonable level but don't need very tight control because their probable life span is shorter than the time it takes to develop complications. Their treatment can be kept very simple. The insulin is being used to keep them 'out of trouble', not to prevent long-term complications.

Finally, people with type 2 diabetes who truly need to be on insulin often find once they have taken the plunge to start insulin that they feel much better and it was actually a good thing to have made the change.

People with Diabetes Shouldn't Exercise

If any myth is really damaging to people with diabetes, it is this one: People with diabetes shouldn't exercise. The truth is exactly the opposite. Exercise is a major component of good diabetes management, one that, unfortunately, all too often gets the least time and effort on the part of the person with diabetes as well as care providers.

Of course, if you have certain complications like haemorrhaging in your eye or severe neuropathy, you need to take precautions or not exercise at all for a time. Certainly, if you're older than 40 and have not exercised, you need to start gradually. Except for these and a few other reasons (refer to Chapter 12), exercise ought to be done regularly by every person with diabetes.

And we're not just talking about aerobic exercise where your heart is beating faster. Some form of muscle strengthening also needs to be a part of your lifestyle. (Refer to Chapter 12 to find out the benefits of muscle strengthening.)

If you have a muscle that you can move, move it!

Getting Life and Health Insurance Is Impossible

In Chapter 19 we show you that you *can* get life and health insurance. Because the insurance industry recognises that people with diabetes take better care of themselves than the general population does, it is more and more willing to insure them. Some unenlightened insurance companies still exist, but most are seeing the light as the vital statistics of the population with diabetes improve. However, life and travel insurance premiums are likely to be higher if you have diabetes.

Private health insurance to supplement your Medicare-funded diabetes care may be beneficial for some people with diabetes. For example, if you have (or someone in your family has) type 1 diabetes, you may want the option of purchasing an insulin pump in the future. Or you may be concerned about public hospital waiting lists for procedures such as heart bypasses or knee replacements.

You may need to shop around to find the health insurance scheme that best suits your needs, but the price should be no higher than what anyone else is paying.

Most Diabetes Is Inherited

Although type 2 diabetes runs in families, type 1 diabetes more often occurs as an isolated event in a family rather than being handed down from parent to child. (Chapter 3 explains why this is the case.) Even type 2 diabetes doesn't come out in every family member. Whether you develop type 2 diabetes or not can depend on such things as body weight, level of activity and other factors.

Occasionally, type 1 diabetes pops up in multiple extended family members, but this is uncommon. If you are a member of a 'cluster' family, the diabetes researchers would be really interested in meeting you all because it's through families with lots of type 1 diabetes that we may learn more about why it develops — and maybe eventually find a cure. If you are interested in being involved in research, discuss this with your diabetes care team or with the Juvenile Diabetes Research Foundation (see Chapter 24 for website details).

Parents should not feel guilty or blame themselves if their child or adolescent develops diabetes. Feeling guilty only makes caring for and living with your child with diabetes even harder. Refer to Chapter 13 for tips on dealing with feelings of guilt, anger or frustration, and for guidance on seeking expert help if these feelings become too difficult to deal with.

Diabetes Wrecks Your Sense of Humour

While at first you may not feel like laughing, after the initial stages of accepting diabetes your sense of humour should return. If your humour doesn't return, it's no laughing matter, so seek some expert help. (Refer to Chapter 13 for more on dealing with diabetes.)

The saying goes, 'Someday, we'll laugh about this'. The question is, 'Why wait?'

Chapter 24

Ten Types of Websites to Learn More about Diabetes

In This Chapter

▶ Checking the general diabetes sites in Australia and around the world

▶ Finding websites with information specific to type 1 diabetes

▶ Exploring websites for young people with diabetes

▶ Browsing for diabetes-friendly nutritional advice

▶ Finding information on exercising safely with diabetes

▶ Seeking online help with mental health issues

▶ Searching for articles and research on medical databases

▶ Looking up information on diabetes-associated health complications

▶ Seeking advice on medications

*1*n just over a decade, the World Wide Web has gone from having little or no information to having more than anyone can digest. This chapter lists the best sites on diabetes: You should be able to get answers to just about any questions that you have, but you must be cautious about the source of the advice. Don't make any major changes in your diabetes care without checking with your GP. In Chapter 21, you find advice about how to differentiate between useful and useless information on the Web — remember that sometimes free advice is worth no more than you pay for it.

The Web is constantly changing and growing. These addresses are valid at the date of publication but they may change at some future date.

General Sites

These sites tell you about diabetes from A to Z. They run the gamut from well-known organisations to individual doctors who specialise in diabetes. Sometimes the sites get a little technical. That is when you need to return to this book for clarification.

- **Australian Diabetes Council:** Previously known as Diabetes Australia NSW. Provides information about all aspects of diabetes. www.australiandiabetescouncil.com.au

- **Australian Diabetes Educators Association:** This is the official website of the organisation representing diabetes educators in Australia. They have a 'Find a Credentialled Diabetes Educator' function to help you access experienced health care professionals to assist you in your management of diabetes. www.adea.com.au

- **Australian Diabetes in Pregnancy Society:** This site is very useful for anyone who diagnosed with gestational diabetes. www.adips.org.au

- **Australian Diabetes Society (ADS):** This is the group that represents endocrinologists and allied health professionals with an interest in diabetes. www.diabetessociety.com.au

- **Australian Indigenous Health Infonet:** This site provides information on many health issues pertinent to indigenous Australians, including diabetes. www.healthinfonet.ecu.edu.au

- **Australian Institute of Health and Welfare (AIHW):** This is Australia's national agency for health and welfare statistics and information. Look here to find out more about statistics related to diabetes in Australia. www.aihw.gov.au

- **The Baker IDI Heart and Diabetes Institute:** This Victorian-based institute is the largest diabetes clinic in Australia. Its huge site presents extensive information for both the general public and health professionals, covering aspects of living with diabetes, as well as a test to determine whether you are at risk of having diabetes, called the Australian Type 2 Diabetes Risk Assessment Tool. www.bakeridi.edu.au

- **Coeliac Society:** This is the site for those who have also been diagnosed with coeliac disease. This is an extremely informative site with lots of information on the gluten-free diet and the contact details of gluten-free restaurants. General information about coeliac disease is also provided. Their excellent quarterly magazine is available to all members. www.coeliacsociety.com.au

- **Department of Health and Ageing:** The federal government health website. General information about diabetes is available, as well as Australian Government programs and statistics. www.health.gov.au

✔ **Diabetes Australia:** Diabetes Australia is an organisation with branches in all states and territories except NSW. They represent people with diabetes, research organisations, doctors and other health professionals involved with diabetes. The national site gives an overview of the services that Diabetes Australia offers and the research that it supports, in addition to facts about diabetes, frequently asked questions, an extensive list of products that are available and local branch addresses. It also provides links to state and territory branches. www.diabetesaustralia.com.au

✔ **Federation of Ethnic Communities Council Australia:** Helpful advice for those for whom English is a second language. www.fecca.org.au

✔ **Garvan Institute:** This site gives an outline of the Diabetes and Metabolism Research Program, which primarily focuses on studying the links between exercise, fat and type 2 diabetes prevention. (Enter the title of this program into the search function on the site to find out more.) You can also find details here of research being done at the Garvan on the genetics of type 1 diabetes. www.garvan.org.au

✔ **Medicare:** The Australian government health provider. Provides details of Medicare-funded services for people with diabetes. www.medicareaustralia.gov.au

✔ **National Aboriginal Community Controlled Health Organisation:** Health information specifically targeted at the Indigenous community. www.naccho.org.au

✔ **National Health and Medical Research Council (NHMRC):** The peak Australian organisation supporting health and medical research. www.nhmrc.gov.au

✔ **Royal Australian College of General Practitioners (RACGP):** The organisation representing your local doctor. Find information on services available and guidelines for management of diabetes. www.racgp.org.au

Type 1 Diabetes

The following sites are specifically related to all aspects of type 1 diabetes.

✔ **Juvenile Diabetes Research Foundation:** The Juvenile Diabetes Research Foundation Australia site contains individual state and territory event calendars (fundraising events, diabetes camps, support groups and seminars), access to *Update* magazine and news and links specifically focusing on children's needs. www.jdrf.org.au

✔ **Reality Check:** This site is produced by a Melbourne-based group of young people with diabetes. It includes access to a unique chat room, which enables young adults to have informal discussions with others about living with diabetes. There are also interactive seminars organised with diabetes specialists. www.realitycheck.org.au

Young People with Diabetes

The sites listed in this section are designed to provide information about diabetes in children and adolescents. The first two are health professional websites and the last one is especially designed for young people with diabetes and their carers.

✔ **Australasian Paediatric Endocrine Group (APEG):** A professional group representing doctors and allied health workers interested in diabetes in the paediatric population. www.apeg.org.au

✔ **International Society for Pediatric and Adolescent Diabetes (ISPAD):** This is a professional organisation that aims to promote research, education and advocacy in childhood and adolescent diabetes. www.ispad.org

✔ **Kids and Teens:** This site has been designed to appeal to kids and is very interactive. It also has information for parents and carers, schools and health professionals. www.diabeteskidsandteens.com.au

Nutrition

The sites listed here range over a wide area and can provide information on the technical aspects of nutrition as well as the practical requirements of eating, like recipes!

✔ **Calorie King:** Commercial website where you can find vast quantities of information on the nutritional value of Australian foods. The site is free to use and also has recipes. www.calorieking.com.au

✔ **Dietitians Association of Australia:** This site provides information relating to the Association's mission statement: 'Better Food, Better Health, Better Living'. Reviews of seminar presentations are available, as well as scientific papers and abstracts relating to the role of diet in diabetes. www.daa.asn.au

✔ **Foods Standards Australia and New Zealand:** The Australian Government website containing the official nutritional values of Australian foods. www.foodstandards.gov.au

✔ **Glycaemic Index:** This is the official Australian glycaemic index site and is linked with the Glycaemic Index Symbol program from the University of Sydney. www.glycemicindex.com

✔ **Nutrition Australia:** A good site for information about the dietary requirements of diabetes. www.nutritionaustralia.org

✔ **Symply Too Good:** This site provides great recipes that are easy and delicious. www.symplytoogood.com.au

Exercise

The following sites provide information about how to exercise safely with diabetes.

✔ **Exercise and Sports Science Australia:** This is the professional body representing exercise physiologists. www.essa.org.au

✔ **Exercise with type 1 diabetes:** This site is run by Alan Bolton, who has type 1 diabetes, and is an elite athlete, exercise physiologist and diabetes educator! The site provides lots of great information for the more serious sportsperson who has type 1 diabetes. www.ext1d.com.au

✔ **Fitness 2 Live:** Aimed mostly at the corporate market, this site also has advice for individuals in both diet and exercise. www.fitness2live.com.au

✔ **HypoActive:** This site was set up by people with type 1 diabetes who wanted to help others become more active. HypoActive offers online support through the site, and their mission statement is to 'inspire and enable the type 1 community to live a more physically active lifestyle'. www.hypoactive.org

✔ **University of NSW Lifestyle and Strength Clinic:** This site provides information on lifestyle and physical activity services. www.lifestyleclinic.net.au

Mental Health

The sites listed in this section cover a wide variety of topics within the mental health area. Although not all are specific to diabetes, much helpful information can be found at the following sites.

- ✔ **Australian Psychological Society:** Use this site to find a psychologist who is qualified to help you. www.psychology.org.au
- ✔ **Beyond Blue:** This organisation provides information about depression to consumers, carers and health professionals. www.beyondblue.org.au
- ✔ **Black Dog Institute:** This institute is an educational, research and clinical facility offering specialist expertise in mood disorders such as bipolar and depression. The institute is a not-for-profit organisation and is oriented towards consumers. www.blackdoginstitute.org.au
- ✔ **Diabetes Counselling Online:** This website is designed for all people living with diabetes, their families and friends. A link is provided to their secure private email counselling service. You can also chat online in a public forum. www.diabetescounselling.com.au
- ✔ **Lifeline Australia:** Lifeline provides services in suicide prevention, crisis support and mental health support. www.lifeline.org.au
- ✔ **SANE Australia:** This is a national charity helping people affected by mental illness. www.sane.org

International Sites

Starting with the Aussie sites is a good idea, but you may wish to see what is happening overseas. Aspects relating to your diabetes management, such as health systems, foods, drugs and equipment vary from country to country, so you may find information on these sites that is different to what is available in Australia. Refer any questions about items you find here to your diabetes care team.

- ✔ **The American Diabetes Association:** This site has just about everything you need to know about diabetes. It is the premier site for diabetes information and has links to other worldwide sites. www.diabetes.org
- ✔ **Children with Diabetes:** This site is the creation of an American father of a child with diabetes and has an enormous database of information for the parents of children with diabetes. It includes the latest research on juvenile diabetes from around the world, virtual online support groups and recipes. www.childrenwithdiabetes.com

- **The Diabetes Monitor:** The Diabetes Monitor is the creation of diabetes specialist Dr William Quick. He discusses every aspect of diabetes, including the latest discoveries, and is continuously monitoring the internet for new, up-to-the minute diabetes information. www.diabetesmonitor.com

- **The International Diabetes Federation:** This organisation of knowledgeable diabetes experts from over 100 countries meets every three years. This website has information and links about all aspects of diabetes for those living with diabetes as well as the health professionals who care for them. www.idf.org

Medical Literature Databases

You can find numerous articles about diabetes from medical publications using these two sites. They are easy to use and give you (for free) a large number of the latest scientific papers on any medical topic of interest.

- **Medscape:** This database is from the United States. www.medscape.com/diabetes-endocrinology

- **PubMed:** This site is provided by the American National Library of Medicine. It is a free digital archive of biomedical and life sciences journal literature. www.ncbi.nlm.nih.gov/PubMed

Diabetes Complications

Many services are available to help people with diabetes who are unfortunate enough to suffer from some of the complications of diabetes. Here we list the most helpful of the major sites.

- **Australasian Podiatry Council:** This site provides foot health tips for people with diabetes. www.apodc.com.au

- **Blind Citizens of Australia:** This site provides contact details for Australia-wide associations, libraries and centres for the blind and visually impaired, as well as access to 'New Horizons', a 15-minute weekly program played on the internet with information on visual impairment issues, current affairs, TV dramas, interviews and sport. www.bca.org.au

- **Kidney Health Australia:** Helpful advice for those who are also suffering from kidney disease. www.kidney.org.au

- **National Heart Foundation:** This site provides extensive information related to heart disease. www.heartfoundation.com.au

- **National Stroke Foundation Australia:** This site provides help and advice for those people who have suffered a stroke, and their carers. www.strokefoundation.com.au

- **Vision Australia:** This site provides help with services for the visually impaired, and links to many associated sites. www.visionaustralia.org.au

Medications Advice

Want to know more about the medicines you take? The following is a comprehensive list of the websites that can best assist you in your quest.

- **Health Insite:** A general website covering all aspects of health. Also has comprehensive links to other reputable websites. www.healthinsite.gov.au

- **National Diabetes Services Scheme:** You can use this site to find your nearest NDSS outlet. www.ndss.com.au

- **Pharmaceutical Benefits Scheme:** For more information on the medicines that are subsidised by the Australian government. www.health.gov.au/pbs

- **Therapeutic Goods Administration:** The TGA regulates both the approval of medicines and medical appliances (such as insulin pumps) in Australia. www.tga.gov.au

Part VII
Appendixes

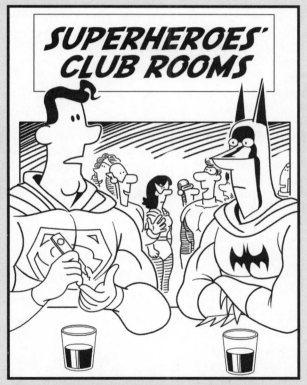

*'I can control my diabetes well enough ...
the toughest bit is trying to do a
finger-prick test when you've
got impenetrable skin.'*

In this part ...

Still want to know more? This part provides information on some specific topics relating to diabetes. We give you more information on insulin pumps, helping you decide whether this might be the right choice for you or your child. We also provide some more practical help to improve your mental health, in the form of mindfulness and relaxation exercises. And if you need to check what a term means, you can flick straight to the handy glossary.

Appendix A

Insulin Pumps

- -

In This Appendix

▶ Learning the basic workings of insulin pumps

▶ Taking the advantages and disadvantages of using pumps into account

▶ Working out whether an insulin pump is the best choice for you

▶ Looking at options available in Australia

- -

*T*he popularity of using an insulin pump or continuous subcutaneous insulin infusions (CSII) to deliver insulin has grown significantly over the years; however, its use is still in its infancy in many areas of Australia. For example, it is quite common for paediatric diabetes services to now offer pump therapy as a first option for delivering insulin rather than via an insulin pen. However this option may not be offered by all adult diabetes services. This may be because of lack of demand or because the hospital or diabetes centre has insufficient staff to provide this service. Providing a pump service requires a large time commitment from a highly skilled diabetes care team — as well as from the person with diabetes.

Pumping is also not for everyone and you should not feel pressured into having a pump if you do not think it's for you!

In this appendix, we cover some of the basic issues regarding pump use that may help you to decide if this is a treatment option for you. For more information on insulin pumps and services available in Australia, consult your diabetes care team.

Understanding How Insulin Pumps Work

An insulin pump is a small battery-powered, computerised pump that's about the size of a pager. The pump holds rapid-acting insulin in a reservoir and then delivers the insulin through an infusion set. If using a continuous glucose monitoring system (CGMS), the system can transmit information directly to the insulin pump and, in some cases, the pump will react accordingly. (Refer to Chapter 9 for more on CGMSs and to Chapter 10 for more on the parts that make up an insulin pump and how it is attached.)

The insulin pump delivers insulin in exact amounts — as small as 0.025 units of insulin per hour! The insulin is delivered in two ways:

- ✔ **Basal** is a small amount of insulin delivered continuously, based on individual needs. The basal rate assists to keep the glucose levels in the target range between meals and/or overnight, so once these basal rates have been set they will need to be finetuned with growth or changes in routine. Your basal insulin requirements vary across the day, and requirements differ between people. Pumps can accommodate these individual variations more effectively than one or two long-acting insulin doses, which deliver insulin at the same level across the day.

    You can set a temporary basal rate on your insulin pump when you exercise, are unwell, or to take into account menstrual cycles and changes in routines.

- ✔ **Bolus** is the insulin taken for meals. The amount taken may be pre-programmed (for example, for children at school) but is usually programmed in when food is eaten, based on the grams of carbohydrate eaten and the blood glucose level before the meal. A correction bolus is an extra amount of insulin given when the glucose is high.

Keep in mind the following when using an insulin pump:

- ✔ The infusion set and reservoir must be changed every two to three days.

- ✔ The pump can be disconnected from the infusion set for short periods, such as during swimming, exercise and showering.

✔ Insulin pumps are not an artificial pancreas — they aren't fully automatic. You must program the pump to give insulin when you need it, which can be time consuming to learn, but is worth it for better blood glucose control.

✔ Insulin pumps only use rapid-acting insulin.

To work out the insulin dose to program into your pump, you need to test your blood glucose before you eat and enter this result into the pump along with the quantity of carbohydrates that you are eating. The pump will calculate how much insulin is to be given, based on information your diabetes care team has entered into the pump. (Refer to Chapter 9 for more on testing your blood glucose levels.)

Members of your diabetes care team are the best people to talk to about what pumps may be suitable for you. They will also help you set your required basal and boluses rates, insulin-to-carbohydrate ratios and correction formulas, according to your individual needs.

Even when using a pump, you must still carry insulin pens with you and be prepared to use them if you have two unexplained high glucose levels in a row.

Looking at the Benefits and Challenges

The benefits of using an insulin pump include the following:

✔ **Accurate dosing.** Insulin delivery is exact and matched to each individual's needs. This accuracy makes it easier to manage growth spurts, sleeping in, hypoglycaemia and illness.

✔ **Flexibility.** Since rapid -acting insulin is used, there is no long-acting insulin waiting to be absorbed. This provides flexibility in timing of exercise and meals and helps you manage on unpredictable days.

✔ **Less severe hypoglycaemia.** More predictable and more precise insulin delivery makes the risk of severe hypoglycaemia less likely.

✔ **Predictability.** Using only rapid -acting insulin means the absorption of insulin is more predictable.

The challenges of using an insulin pump include the following:

- **Body image and psychological adjustment:** Some people don't like the idea of being attached to a device all the time.

- **Education:** A lot of preparation is required before pump therapy can be commenced and to ensure you take advantage of the pump's many features.

- **Hypoglycaemia:** Tighter control of blood glucose levels can lead to more lows.

- **Risk of diabetic ketoacidosis (DKA):** This can happen because no long-acting insulin is present in the body, so any interruption of insulin delivery — caused by, for example, a kink in the line carrying the insulin — will cause the glucose levels to rise quickly.

Is an Insulin Pump Right for You?

Studies have shown that after starting an insulin pump most patients experience much better blood glucose control and a lower HbA1c. However, over time this improvement tends to wear off and blood glucose levels often return to pre-pump levels. The reason for this is probably related to the rather intensive support you usually get when first going onto the pump, and the inevitable loss of motivation to keep counting carbohydrate and adjusting insulin for variations in activity as time goes on!

For many people, however, going onto a pump is more to do with its effect on their lifestyle. The following groups of people often find a pump is the best option for them:

- Those who don't want to have to worry about forgetting their insulin

- Small children, whose insulin requirements are often very small

- Women who require very tight blood glucose control in preparation for a pregnancy

- Shift workers or others whose unusual working hours often make using multiple injections difficult or impractical

- People who have hypoglycaemia unawareness

If you think an insulin pump is right for you, you need to work closely with your diabetes care team to learn how to use the pump and commit to follow-up care and education.

Insulin pumps cost between $5,000 and $8,000. If you have private health insurance, the full cost will be covered by your fund at a replacement rate of one pump every five years. Government subsidies are also available for carers of children under 18 years of age. The family must be eligible for Medicare and not have access to private health insurance. The infusion sets are subsidised through the NDSS scheme, but still cost approximately $40 per month.

Finding Out More

If you think an insulin pump might be a good choice for you, talk to your diabetes care team to find out more about the options available in Australia. You can also go directly to the manufacturers' websites, to give you an idea of what's available and the features of each system before talking more with your care team.

In Australia, four companies provide insulin pumps. These companies, as well as their website details, are as follows:

- ✔ Accu-Chek Spirit Insulin Pump accuchek.com.au/au/products/insulinpumps/index.html
- ✔ Animas Insulin Pump www.amsl.com.au/products/
- ✔ Dana Insulin Pump www.diabetesnsw.com.au/
- ✔ Medtronic Insulin Pumps www.medtronic-diabetes.com.au/

Appendix B

Mental Health Exercises

To help you care for your mental health when living with diabetes, this appendix outlines some strategies to calm your body and mind. For many people, worries and distressing thoughts can lead to stress and feelings of anxiety or depression. When you're under stress, your body goes through changes, including muscles contracting and becoming tense.

Mindfulness and relaxation are two different approaches to calming your body and mind. Mindfulness focuses on 'observing' your thoughts, feelings and sensations, rather than challenging them. Relaxation, on the other hand, works to counter the physical changes that go along with stress, such as relaxing your muscles, and to distract your mind from worries.

Try these simple techniques and see what works best for you. Remember that both mindfulness and relaxation take practice. Choose the exercises that you prefer and try to use them every day. Remember, the more often you practice, the greater the benefits!

Mindfulness Exercises

Mindfulness is all about purposefully paying attention to the unfolding experience. It has been cultivated through several forms of meditation derived from Buddhist meditative practices and is a skill that can be developed with practice.

Although mindfulness interventions may result in relaxation, they are not designed as relaxation techniques. In contrast to cognitive behaviour therapy (refer to Chapter 13), mindfulness training does not aim to change thought content. Rather, mindfulness approaches are based on direct observation of the changing nature of thoughts, feelings and sensations as a way of 'being' rather than as a therapeutic problem-solving technique.

Over the past 30 years, a growing number of therapeutic interventions have been developed that utilise mindfulness as a key component in the treatment of medical illness, particular chronic illness such as diabetes, chronic pain and affective disorders, where acceptance of the symptoms and an overall sense of greater empowerment and ability to put emotional distance between the person and their symptoms have been found to be very useful.

The best way of explaining mindfulness is to experience it. Go ahead and try the simple exercises that follow — you will be amazed how good they makes you feel. (For even more help with mindfulness, see *Mindfulness For Dummies* by Shamash Alidina (Wiley Publishing Ltd).)

A one-minute introduction to mindfulness

You can start with this simple one minute exercise. Have a go — it makes you feel great. Here's how:

- ✔ Sit in front of a clock or watch so you can time the passing of one minute.

- ✔ Focus your entire attention on your breathing — and nothing else — for the whole minute.

Don't put it off — have a go now and find a minute per day to practice.

Taking a body scan

The 'body scan' is another mindfulness technique and can be achieved by working through the following:

- ✔ Take a few moments to feel your body as a whole, from head to toe, then the envelope of your skin, the sensations where your skin touches your clothes, and anything else.

- ✔ Bring your attention to the toes of your left foot. Direct your breathing towards them (visualising that your breath is travelling from your nose to your foot and back).

✔ Allow yourself to feel any sensation from your toes. If you feel nothing, allow this too.

✔ Stay with this until you are ready to repeat the process with your forefoot, sole, ankle, leg and thigh. Then start the same process over with the toes of your right foot.

✔ Move to your lower belly, lower back, upper belly, upper back, shoulder, arm, elbow, forearm, hand fingers, neck, face and head. Include more body parts if you wish.

Initially practice this body scan exercise for 10 to 15 minutes once or twice daily. Aim to build up to 10 to 45 minutes twice daily, or as much as you feel benefits you.

Once you're comfortable with the body scan exercise and your mind settles into the process, the whole body scan can take between 30 and 45 minutes. If you don't have this much time on any particular day, you can modify the process to only scan some body parts. You will still feel the benefits, even with a shorter session.

After practising for the allotted time, gently move back into the activities that await you.

Starting with mindful breathing helps to orient yourself to your body. You can then move onto other mindful practices, such as mindfulness of eating or mindfulness of walking, or you may choose to stay with the breath.

Mindfulness of walking

When walking in a mindful way, focus all of your attention on your experience of walking — don't try to do anything else at the same time, such as listening to music or eating.

Consider the following when adopting mindfulness of walking:

✔ Start with just a few minutes of mindful walking. You can then build up to longer periods.

✔ While walking, concentrate on the feel of the ground under your feet, your breathing while walking and your surroundings in the present. Feel the temperature on your skin, the sensation of the wind or air, the smells around you, the sights of the sky and trees.

✔ If you find any thoughts coming into your mind (such as thoughts about where you are going or what you are going to do), simply acknowledge that a thought came into your mind, let the thought go and bring your attention back to your walking.

Mindfulness of eating

The same principles used in mindfulness of walking (refer to previous section) apply to mindfulness of eating: Focus all of your attention on your experiences while eating. You can start off with choosing a small, simple piece of food to eat in a mindful way, such as a sultana. You can then try eating a whole meal mindfully.

Consider the following when adopting mindfulness of eating:

✔ Sit down at a table with your food. Do not do anything else while eating mindfully — don't listen to music, watch television, read a newspaper or talk.

✔ Pay full attention to the piece of food you select to eat — how you cut the food, how it smells, the shape and colours of the food.

✔ Slowly chew each mouthful, paying attention to the muscles you use to chew, the texture and the taste of the food.

✔ If you find any thoughts coming into your mind, let the thoughts go and bring your attention back to the food.

Not only will eating mindfully help you purposefully pay attention to the present moment, but you may also be amazed at how different food tastes when eaten in this way and how filling a meal can be.

Relaxation Exercises

Stress is known to have an effect on the onset and course of diabetes. A relaxation exercise is any method or activity that promotes a state of increased calmness. Usually, it is used to reduce levels of anxiety, stress or anger but it is wise to practice relaxation exercises when you are already feeling calm, so that the exercises are available when needed.

Relaxation exercises can be used alone or as part of a broader stress management program and can decrease muscle tension, lower blood pressure and blood sugar levels, and slow heart and breath rates, as well as providing other health benefits. A wide variety of relaxation exercises are available — the trick is finding some that suit you.

In this section, we provide some simple relaxation exercises. You may need to practice these a few times to get used to them and make sure the process behind them is cemented in your mind. Try each of the exercises provided and rate them all as *Would use again*, *May use again* or *Would not use again*. Then chose the one(s) that work best for you.

Try the following exercises:

- **Whole body tension:** Tense everything in your whole body; stay with that tension. Hold it as long as you can without feeling pain. Slowly release the tension, feeling it as it leaves your body very gradually. Repeat three times.

- **Imagining air as a cloud:** Open your imagination and focus on your breathing. As your breathing becomes calm and regular, imagine that the air comes to you as a cloud — it fills you and goes out. You may imagine the cloud to be a particular colour.

- **Picking a spot to focus on:** With your head level and body relaxed, pick a spot to focus on (eyes open at this point). When ready, count five breaths backward and allow your eyes to gradually close with each breath. Concentrate on each breath. When you get to 'one', your eyes will be closed. Focus on your feelings of relaxation.

- **Counting ten breaths backward:** Allow yourself to feel at ease. Count each breath slowly from ten to one. With each count, allow yourself to feel heavier and more relaxed. With each exhale, allow the tension to leave your body.

- **Reimagining images of stress:** This exercise suits people who like visualisation techniques. Look at Table B-1 and choose one of the images on the left side, that you feel best represents you when you are feeling tense. Next, imagine the process of your body slowly relaxing and becoming like the image on the right side of the table. Feel each part of your body loosening, relaxing and looking like the new image — for example, feel the 'knots' in your neck and shoulders 'loosening' and relaxing and so on.

Table B-1   Tips for Reimagining Stressful Images

When you think of images like	Imagine instead
Tight knots of rope	Knots loosening
Feel of icy wind	Wind becoming gentle, mild breeze
Red, tense muscles	Red muscles softening and turning blue or lightening to pink
Block of ice	Ice melting in the sun to warm water

Glossary

advanced glycosylation (glycated) end products (AGEs): Chemical combinations of *glucose* with other substances in the body. Too much may damage various organs.

alpha cells: Cells in the Islets of Langerhans within the *pancreas* that make *glucagon*, which raises blood glucose.

amino acids: Compounds that link together to form proteins.

amyotrophy: A form of diabetic *neuropathy* causing muscle wasting and weakness.

angiography: Using a dye injected into the bloodstream to take pictures of blood vessels to detect disease. In diabetes, angiography is often used in the eyes and coronary arteries.

antibodies: Substances formed when the body detects something foreign such as bacteria or viruses.

antigens: Substances against which *antibodies* form.

atherosclerosis (arteriosclerosis): Narrowing of arteries due to deposits of cholesterol and other factors. Can occur in the heart (cardiovascular disease), in the brain (cerebrovascular disease) or in the legs (peripheral vascular disease).

autoimmune disorder: Disease in which the body's immune system mistakenly attacks its own tissues.

autonomic neuropathy: Diseases of nerves that affect organs not under conscious control, such as the heart, intestine and blood vessels.

background retinopathy: An early stage of diabetic eye involvement that does not reduce vision.

beta cells: Cells in the Islets of Langerhans in the *pancreas*, which make the key hormone insulin.

body mass index: A number derived by dividing the weight (in kilograms) by the height times the height (in metres). Used to determine the category of weight (either underweight, normal, overweight or obese).

carbohydrate: One of the three major energy sources. Carbohydrate is found in grains, fruits and starchy vegetables and is responsible for raising the blood glucose.

carbohydrate counting: Estimating the amount of carbohydrate in food in order to determine insulin needs.

cataract: A clouding of the lens of the eye often found earlier and more commonly in people with diabetes.

cerebrovascular disease (CVD): A disease of the arteries that supply the brain with blood, carrying oxygen and nutrients.

Charcot's arthropathy (or Charcot's foot): Destruction of joints and soft tissue in the foot leading to an unusable foot as a result of diabetic *neuropathy*.

cholesterol: A form of fat that is needed in the body for production of certain hormones. Can lead to *atherosclerosis* if present in excessive levels.

continuous subcutaneous insulin infusion (CSII): Continuous delivery of insulin under the skin by an *insulin pump*.

creatinine: A substance in blood that is measured to reflect the level of kidney function.

diabetes educator: A nurse who has specialised in diabetes education who can assist people with diabetes to manage their condition.

diabetic ketoacidosis: An acute loss of control of diabetes with high blood glucose levels and breakdown of fat leading to acidification of the blood with nausea, vomiting and dehydration, which can lead to coma and death.

dialysis: Artificial filtering to clean the blood when the kidneys are not working.

dietitian: A health care professional who specialises in nutrition and the use of nutritional approaches to treat disease.

endocrinologist: A doctor who specialises in diseases of the hormone-producing glands, including the adrenal glands, the thyroid, the pituitary, the parathyroid glands, the ovaries, testicles and pancreas.

euglycaemia: A state in which the blood glucose remains in the normal range.

exercise physiologist: A health professional who specialises in the delivery of exercise, lifestyle and behavioural modification programs for the prevention and management of chronic diseases and injuries.

fibre: A substance in plants that can't be digested, so it provides no energy. It can lower fat and blood glucose if it dissolves in water and is absorbed or can help prevent constipation if it does not dissolve in water and remains in the intestine.

gastroparesis: A form of *autonomic neuropathy* involving nerves to the stomach so that food is held for too long in the stomach.

gestational diabetes mellitus: Diabetes that occurs during a pregnancy, usually ending at delivery.

glucagon: A hormone made in the *alpha cells* of the *pancreas* that raises *glucose* and can be injected in severe *hypoglycaemia*.

glucometer: A machine designed to measure blood glucose levels.

glucose: The body's main source of energy in the blood and cells.

glycaemic index: The speed at which a given food raises blood glucose, usually compared to 50 grams of pure glucose. Low glycaemic index foods are preferred in diabetes.

glycogen: The storage form of glucose in the liver and muscles.

glycosuria: Glucose in the urine.

glycosylated (glycated) haemoglobin: *See* **haemoglobin A1c**.

haemoglobin A1c: A measurement of blood glucose control reflecting the average blood glucose for the last 60 to 90 days.

high density lipoprotein (HDL) cholesterol: A particle in blood that carries cholesterol and helps reduce *atherosclerosis*.

honeymoon period: A length of time of variable duration, usually less than a year, after a diagnosis of type 1 diabetes when the need for injections of insulin is reduced or eliminated.

hyperglycaemia: Elevated levels of blood glucose; greater than 7 mmol/L fasting or 7.8 mmol/L after food.

hyperglycaemic hyperosmolar state: Very high glucose in type 2 diabetes associated with severe dehydration but not excessive fat breakdown and acidosis. It can lead to coma and death. Previously known as hyperosmolar non-ketotic state (or HONK).

hyperinsulinaemia: More insulin than normal in the blood, often found early in type 2 diabetes.

hyperlipidaemia: Elevated levels of fat in the blood.

hypoglycaemia: Levels of blood glucose lower than normal, usually less than 4.0 mmol/L. Usually caused by excessive amounts of insulin and/or too much exercise and/or too little food.

impaired fasting glucose (IFG): Levels of glucose between 6.1 and 6.9 mmol/L when in a fasting state. Not normal, but not high enough to be diagnosed as diabetes.

impaired glucose tolerance (IGT): Levels of glucose between 7.8 and 11.1 mmol/L after eating. Not normal but not quite high enough for a diagnosis of diabetes.

impotence: Loss of the ability to have or sustain an erection of the penis.

insulin: The key hormone that controls blood *glucose*; it permits glucose to enter cells and stops the liver overproducing glucose.

insulin pump: Device that slowly delivers insulin through a catheter under the skin throughout a full 24-hour period. It can also be used to give a dose before meals.

insulin resistance: Decreased response to insulin found early in type 2 diabetes.

islet cells: The cells in the *pancreas* that make insulin, *glucagon* and other hormones.

ketoacidosis: Very high levels of blood glucose with large amounts of acid (ketones) in the blood.

ketones: The breakdown products of fat metabolism.

ketonuria: Ketones in the urine.

kilojoule: The unit of measurement of the energy content of food.

lancet: A sharp needle to prick the skin for a blood glucose test.

laser treatment: Using a device that burns tiny areas in the back of the eye to prevent worsening of *retinopathy*.

lipoatrophy (fat atrophy): Indented areas where insulin is constantly injected.

lipohypertrophy (fat hypertrophy): Swelling of the fat under the skin where insulin is constantly injected.

low density lipoprotein (LDL): A particle in the blood containing cholesterol and thought to be responsible for *atherosclerosis*.

macrosomia: Description of a large baby born when the mother's diabetes is not well controlled.

macrovascular complications: Heart attack, stroke or diminished blood flow to the legs.

metabolic syndrome: A combination of hypertension, increased abdominal fat, high *triglycerides*, low HDL cholesterol, often obesity, and high uric acid associated with diabetes and increased heart attacks.

microalbuminuria: Loss of small but abnormal amounts of protein in the urine.

microvascular complications: Eye disease, nerve disease or kidney disease.

monounsaturated fat: One form of fat from vegetable sources like olives and nuts that does not raise cholesterol.

National Diabetes Services Scheme (NDSS): Federal government–funded scheme administered by Diabetes Australia to subsidise the cost of diabetes supplies.

neovascularisation: Formation of new vessels, especially in the *retina* of the eye.

nephropathy: Damage to the kidneys.

neuropathic ulcer: An infected area usually on the leg or foot resulting from damage that was not felt because of *neuropathy*.

neuropathy: Damage to nerves, particularly those carrying sensation in the legs and feet.

ophthalmologist: A doctor who specialises in diseases of the eyes.

oral glucose tolerance test (OGTT): This test can determine the difference between having *prediabetes* and diabetes. It involves fasting overnight, having your blood glucose tested, then drinking a glucose-containing drink, followed by further measurements of your blood glucose levels at one hour and two hours.

oral hypoglycaemic agent: A glucose-lowering drug taken by mouth.

pancreas: The organ behind the stomach that contains the *islet cells*.

periodontal disease: Gum damage, which is more common in uncontrolled diabetes.

podiatrist: A health professional who specialises in treating the feet.

polydipsia: Excessive intake of water or other fluids.

polyunsaturated fat: A form of fat from vegetables that may not raise cholesterol but lowers *high density lipoprotein (HDL) cholesterol*.

polyuria: Excessive urination.

postprandial: After eating.

prediabetes: The term used to describe impaired fasting glucose or impaired glucose tolerance, often the precursors for diabetes.

proliferative retinopathy: Undesirable proliferation of blood vessels in front of the *retina*.

protein: A source of energy for the body made up of amino acids and found in meat, fish, poultry, dairy foods and legumes.

proteinuria: Abnormal loss of protein from the body into the urine.

psychiatrist: A health professional who is first trained as a doctor and then studies for a further five years to specialise in mental health. Treatment methods can be physical, psychological, involve medication, or may be a combination of these approaches.

psychologist: A health professional who is an expert in human behaviour. Scientifically supported and reliable psychological therapies are used to treat individuals and families.

receptor: Places on cells that bind to substances like insulin to permit the substance to do its job.

retina: The part of the eye that senses light.

retinopathy: Disease of the *retina*.

saturated fat: A form of fat from animals that raises cholesterol.

triglycerides: The main form of fat in animals.

visceral fat: The fat accumulation in the abdomen that results in increased waist measurement.

vitrectomy: Surgical removal of the gel in the centre of the eyeball because of blood leakage and the formation of scar tissue.

very low density lipoprotein (VLDL): The main particle in the blood that carries *triglycerides*.

Index

• *Q* •

• *R* •

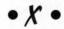

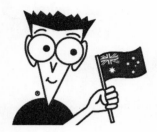

FOR DUMMIES®

Health, Fitness & Pregnancy

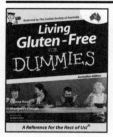

978-0-73140-760-6
$34.95

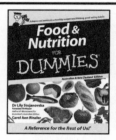

978-0-73140-596-1
$34.95

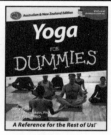

978-1-74031-059-8
$39.95

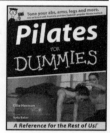

978-1-74031-074-1
$39.95

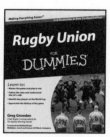

978-0-73037-656-9
$39.95

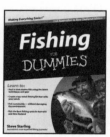

978-1-74216-984-2
$39.95

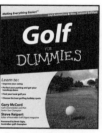

978-0-73037-536-4
$39.95

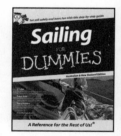

978-0-73140-644-9
$39.95

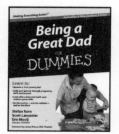

978-1-74216-972-9
$39.95

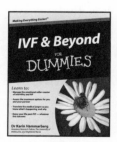

978-1-74216-946-0
$39.95

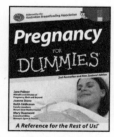

978-1-74031-103-8
$39.95

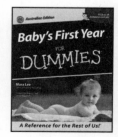

978-1-74031-042-0
$39.95

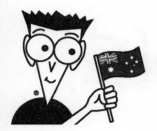

FOR DUMMIES®

Reference

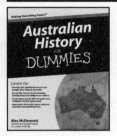

978-1-74216-999-6
$39.95

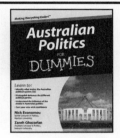

978-1-74216-982-8
$39.95

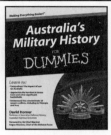

978-1-74216-983-5
$45.00

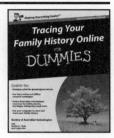

978-0-73140-909-9
$39.95

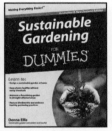

978-1-74216-945-3
$39.95

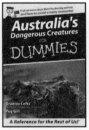

978-0-73140-722-4
$29.95

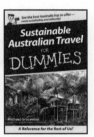

978-0-73140-784-2
$34.95

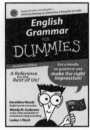

978-0-73140-752-1
$34.95

Technology

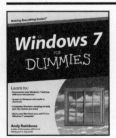

978-0-47049-743-2
$32.95

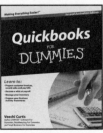

978-1-74246-896-9
$39.95

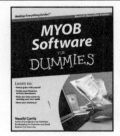

978-1-74216-998-9
$45.00

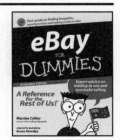

978-1-74031-159-5
$39.95

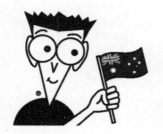

FOR DUMMIES®

Business & Investing

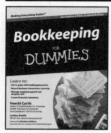

Bookkeeping
FOR DUMMIES

978-1-74216-971-2
$39.95

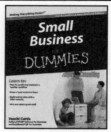

Small Business
FOR DUMMIES

978-1-74216-853-1
$39.95

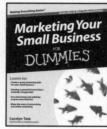

Marketing Your Small Business
FOR DUMMIES

978-1-74216-853-1
$39.95

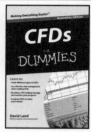

CFDs
FOR DUMMIES

978-1-74216-939-2
$34.95

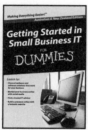

Getting Started in Small Business IT
FOR DUMMIES

978-0-73037-668-2
$19.95

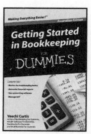

Getting Started in Bookkeeping
FOR DUMMIES

978-1-74246-874-7
$19.95

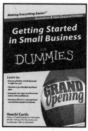

Getting Started in Small Business
FOR DUMMIES

978-1-74216-962-0
$19.95

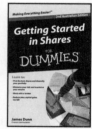

Getting Started in Shares
FOR DUMMIES

978-1-74246-885-3
$19.95

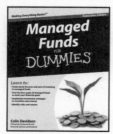

Managed Funds
FOR DUMMIES

978-1-74216-942-2
$39.95

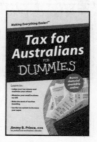

Tax for Australians
FOR DUMMIES

978-1-74246-848-8
$34.95

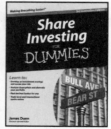

Share Investing
FOR DUMMIES

978-1-74246-889-1
$39.95

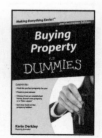

Buying Property
FOR DUMMIES

978-0-73037-556-2
$29.95